The Plant-Based Lunch Recipes Collection

Healthy and Tasty Lunch Recipes to Start Your Plant-Based Diet and Boost Your Lifestyle

Dave Ingram

© **Copyright 2020 - All rights reserved.**

The content contained within this book may not be reproduced, duplicated or transmitted without direct written permission from the author or the publisher.

Under no circumstances will any blame or legal responsibility be held against the publisher, or author, for any damages, reparation, or monetary loss due to the information contained within this book. Either directly or indirectly.

Legal Notice:

This book is copyright protected. This book is only for personal use. You cannot amend, distribute, sell, use, quote or paraphrase any part, or the content within this book, without the consent of the author or publisher.

Disclaimer Notice:

Please note the information contained within this document is for educational and entertainment purposes only. All effort has been executed to present accurate, up to date, and reliable, complete information. No warranties of any kind are declared or implied. Readers acknowledge that the author is not engaging in the rendering of legal, financial, medical or professional advice. The content within this book has been derived from various sources. Please consult a licensed professional before attempting any techniques outlined in this book.

By reading this document, the reader agrees that under no circumstances is the author responsible for any losses, direct or indirect, which are incurred as a result of the use of information contained within this document, including, but not limited to, — errors, omissions, or inaccuracies.

Table of contents

Loaded Kale Salad 5

Black Bean and Quinoa Salad 7

Garden Pasta Salad 9

Roasted Vegetables and Tofu Salad 11

Farro and Lentil Salad 13

Greek Zoodle Bowl 15

Pesto Quinoa with White Beans 17

Green Bean Casserole 19

Pumpkin Risotto 21

Brown Rice and Vegetable Stir-Fry 23

Spicy Sesame & Edamame Noodles 25

Quick & Easy Tomato and Herb Gigantes Beans 27

Creamy Vegan Spinach Pasta 29

Vegan Bake Pasta with Bolognese Sauce and Cashew Cream 31

5 Ingredients Pasta 34

Sabich Sandwich 36

Tofu and Pesto Sandwich 38

Chickpea and Mayonnaise Salad Sandwich 40

Tahini Broccoli 42

Steamed Cauliflower 43

Cauliflower Tacos 45

Sweet Potatoes 47

Smoky Meal 49

Roasted Vegetables and Quinoa Bowls 50

Sweet Potato and Quinoa Bowl 53

- Chickpea Salad Bites ... 55
- Avocado and Chickpeas Lettuce Cups ... 57
- Pappardelle with Cavolo Nero (cabbage) & Walnut Sauce ... 59
- Veggie Sausage & Sun-Dried Tomato One Pot Pasta ... 61
- Chickpea Sunflower Sandwich ... 63
- Stir Fry Noodles ... 65
- Spicy Sweet Chili Veggie Noodles ... 67
- Creamy Vegan Mushroom Pasta ... 70
- Vegan Chinese Noodles ... 73
- Vegetable Penne Pasta ... 76
- Chestnut Mushroom Bourguignon ... 78
- Broad Bean, Fennel & Baby Carrot Pilaf ... 80
- Spelled Spaghetti with Avocado Pesto ... 82
- Mushrooms Sandwich ... 84
- Rainbow Taco Boats ... 86
- Eggplant Sandwich ... 88
- Lentil, Cauliflower and Grape Salad ... 90
- Spaghetti in Spicy Tomato Sauce ... 93
- 20 Minutes Vegetarian Pasta ... 96
- Creamy Vegan Pumpkin Pasta ... 98
- Loaded Creamy Vegan Pesto Pasta ... 100
- Mediterranean Pizza ... 102
- Red Lentil and Chickpea Bowl ... 104
- Curry Wraps ... 106
- One Pan Spicy Rice ... 108

Loaded Kale Salad

Preparation Time: 10 minutes

Cooking Time: 30 minutes

Servings: 4

Ingredients:

1 ½ cup cooked quinoa

For The Vegetables:

1 whole beet, peeled, sliced

4 large carrots, peeled, chopped 1/2 teaspoon curry powder

1/8 teaspoon sea salt

2 tablespoons melted coconut oil For The Dressing:

¼ teaspoon of sea salt

2 tablespoons maple syrup 3 tablespoons lemon juice 1/3 cup tahini

1/4 cup water For the Salad:

1/2 cup sprouts

1 medium avocado, peeled, pitted, cubed 1/2 cup chopped cherry tomatoes

8 cups chopped kale 1/4 cup hemp seeds

Directions:

1. Set the oven it to 375 degrees F and let it preheat.

2. Take a baking sheet, place beets and carrots on it, drizzle with oil, season with curry powder and salt, toss until coated, and then bake for 30 minutes until tender and golden brown.

3. Place all the ingredients in it and whisk until well combined, set aside until required.

4. Assemble the salad and for this, take a large salad bowl, place kale leaves in it, add remaining ingredients for the salad along with roasted vegetables, drizzle with prepared dressing and toss until combined.

5. Serve straight away.

Nutrition: 472 Cal 22.8 g Fat 3.8 g Saturated Fat 58.7 g Carbohydrates 12.5 g Fiber 9.2 g Sugars 14.6 g Protein;

Black Bean and Quinoa Salad

Preparation Time: 35 minutes

Cooking Time: 20 minutes

Servings: 4

Ingredients:

For the Salad:

1 cup of corn

1 ½ cup cooked black beans 1 cup quinoa

1/2 cup minced red onion

2 medium tomatoes, chopped 4 tablespoons chopped cilantro 2 cups of water

For The Dressing:

4 tablespoons lime juice 2 tablespoons lime zest

¼ teaspoon of sea salt 2 tablespoons olive oil

Directions:
1. Pour in water, add quinoa, and bring it to a boil.
2. Cook the quinoa for 15 minutes.

3.   While quinoa cooks, take a small bowl, place all of its ingredients in it and then whisk until combined, set aside until required.

4.   When quinoa has cooked, fluff it with a fork, then transfer it into a medium bowl and put it in the fridge for 23 minutes.

5.   Add remaining ingredients for the salad into the quinoa, drizzle with the dressing, and then toss until well mixed.

6.   Serve straight away.

Nutrition: 229 Cal 10 g Fat 2 g Saturated Fat 27 g Carbohydrates 3 g Fiber 2 g Sugars 6 g Protein;

Garden Pasta Salad

Preparation Time: 10 minutes

Cooking Time: 12 minutes

Servings: 4

Ingredients:

For the Salad:

1		cup kale

1/4 cup chopped basil

2		cups of sliced yellow cherry tomatoes 16 ounces tri-colored pasta

For the Dressing:

1/2 teaspoon sea salt

¼ teaspoon ground black pepper 1 teaspoon dried Italian seasoning 1/2 cup white wine vinegar

3		tablespoons lemon juice 1 teaspoon olive oil

Directions:

1.	Cook the pasta, and for this, take a large pot half full with salty water, place it over medium heat and bring it to a boil.

2.	Cook pasta for 11 minutes until tender, and then drain well into a colander.

3. While pasta cooks, prepare the dressing, and for this, take a small bowl, place all of its ingredients in it and whisk until combined.

4. Transfer pasta into a large bowl, add remaining ingredients for the salad in it, drizzle with prepared dressing and then toss until well combined.

5. Serve straight away.

Nutrition: 424 Cal 3 g Fat 0 g Saturated Fat 46 g Carbohydrates 5 g Fiber 8 g Sugars 13 g Protein

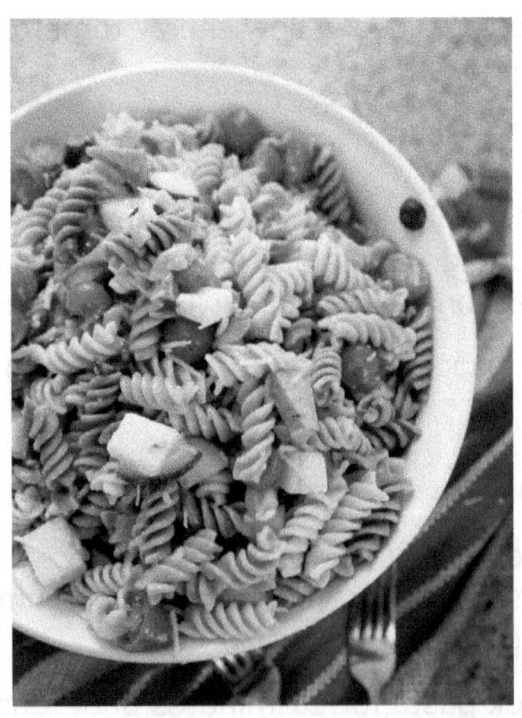

Roasted Vegetables and Tofu Salad

Preparation Time: 10 minutes

Cooking Time: 25 minutes

Servings: 4

Ingredients:

For the salad:

2 cups chopped tofu, firm, pressed, drained 2 cups cooked chickpeas

4 cups spinach

2 cups broccoli floret

2 cups sweet potato, peeled

2 cups Brussel sprout, halved

4 teaspoons ground black pepper 4 teaspoons salt

4 tablespoons red chili powder 1 cup olive oil

For the dressing:

2 teaspoons salt

2 teaspoons ground black pepper 4 teaspoons dried thyme

4 tablespoons lemon juice 4 tablespoons olive oil

2 teaspoons water

½ cup hummus

Directions:

1. Set the oven it to 400 degrees F and let it preheat.

2. Take a large baking sheet, grease it with oil, and spread broccoli florets in one-fifth of the portion, reserving few florets for later use.

3. Add sprouts, sweet potatoes, tofu, and chickpeas as an individual pile on the baking sheet, drizzle with oil, season with salt, black pepper, and red chili powder and then bake for 25 minutes until the tofu has turned nicely golden brown and vegetables are softened, tossing halfway.

4. While vegetables, grains, and tofu are being roasted, prepare the dressing and for this, take a medium jar, add all of its ingredients in it, stir until well combined, and then divide the dressing among four large mason jars.

5. When vegetables, grains, and tofu has been roasted, distribute evenly among four mason jars along with reserved cauliflower florets and shut with lid.

6. When ready to eat, shake the Mason jar until salad is coated with the dressing and then serve.

Nutrition: 477 Cal 24 g Fat 5 g Saturated Fat 52 g Carbohydrates 16 g Fiber

11 g Sugars 21 g Protein;

Farro and Lentil Salad

Preparation Time: 10 minutes

Cooking Time: 0 minutes

Servings: 4

Ingredients:

For the Salad:

1 cup grape tomato, halved

½ cup diced yellow bell pepper

1 cup diced cucumber,

½ cup red bell pepper

1 cup fresh arugula

1/3 cup chopped parsley 1 ½ cups lentils, cooked 3 ½ cups farro, cooked

For the Dressing:

½ teaspoon minced garlic

½ tsp salt

¼ tsp ground black pepper 1 teaspoon Italian seasoning

1 teaspoon Dijon mustard

2 tablespoons red wine vinegar 2 tablespoons lemon juice

1/3 cup olive oil

Directions:

1. Except for arugula, toss the ingredients until combined.

2. Take a bowl, add all of its ingredients, and then stir whisk until well combined.

3. Put the dressing on the salad, toss until well coated, then distribute salad among four bowls and top with arugula.

4. Serve straight away.

Nutrition: 379 Cal 10 g Fat 2 g Saturated Fat 63.5 g Carbohydrates 11 g Fiber 2.5 g Sugars 12.5 g Protein;

Greek Zoodle Bowl

Preparation Time: 10 minutes

Cooking Time: 0 minutes

Servings: 4

Ingredients:

½ cup chopped artichokes 14 cherry tomatoes, chopped

1 medium red bell peppers, cored, chopped 4 medium zucchini

1 medium yellow bell pepper, cored, chopped 6 tablespoons hemp hearts

1 English cucumber

6 tablespoons chopped red onion

2 tbsp chopped parsley leaves 2 tablespoons chopped mint

For the Greek Dressing:

2 tablespoons chopped mint 1 teaspoon garlic powder

½ teaspoon salt

¼ teaspoon dried oregano

2 teaspoons Italian seasoning 3 tablespoons red wine vinegar 1 tablespoon olive oil

Directions:

1. Prepare zucchini and cucumber noodles and for this, spiralize them by using a spiralizer or vegetable peeler and then divide evenly among four bowls.

2. Top zucchini and cucumber noodles with artichokes, tomato, bell pepper, hemp hearts, onion, parsley, and mint, and then set aside until required.

3. Prepare the dressing, take a small bowl, add all the ingredients for the dressing, and whisk until combined.

4. Add the prepared dressing evenly into each bowl, then toss until the vegetables are well coated with the dressing and serve.

Nutrition: 250 Cal 14 g Fat 3 g Saturated Fat 19 g Carbohydrates 5 g Fiber 9 g Sugars 13 g Protein;

Pesto Quinoa with White Beans

Preparation Time: 5 minutes

Cooking Time: 15 minutes

Servings: 4

Ingredients:

12 ounces cooked white bean 3 ½ cups quinoa, cooked

1 medium zucchini, sliced

¾ cup sun-dried tomato

¼ cup pine nuts

1 tablespoon olive oil

For the Pesto:

1/3 cup walnuts 2 cups arugula

1 teaspoon minced garlic 2 cups basil

¾ teaspoon salt

¼ tsp pepper 1 tablespoon lemon juice

1/3 cup olive oil

2 tablespoons water

Directions:

1. Prepare the pesto, and for this, place all of its ingredients in a food processor and pulse for 2 minutes

until smooth, scraping the sides of the container frequently and set aside until required.

2. Add oil and when hot, add zucchini and cook for 4 minutes until tender-crisp.

3. Season zucchini with salt and black pepper, cook for 2 minutes until lightly brown, add tomatoes and white beans and continue cooking for 4 minutes until white beans begin to crisp.

4. Stir in pine nuts, cook for 2 minutes until toasted, then remove the pan from heat and transfer zucchini mixture into a medium bowl.

5. Add quinoa and pesto, stir until well combined, then distribute among four bowls and then serve.

Nutrition: 352 Cal 27.3 g Fat 5 g Saturated Fat 33.7 g Carbohydrates 5.7 g Fiber 4.5 g Sugars 9.7 g Protein;

Green Bean Casserole

Preparation Time: 5 minutes

Cooking Time: 40 minutes

Servings: 4

Ingredients:

6 ounces fried onions

1 ½ cups cremini mushrooms, diced 16 ounces frozen green beans

½ cup diced white onion

1 tablespoon minced garlic

3 ½ tablespoons all-purpose flour 1/3 teaspoon ground black pepper

½ teaspoon dried oregano 3 ½ tablespoons olive oil

2 cups vegetable broth, hot

Directions:

1.   Set the oven to 432 degrees F and let it preheat.

2.   Place a sauceoan over medium heat, add oil, and when hot, add onion and mushrooms, stir in garlic and cook for 4 minutes until tender.

3.   Stir in flour until the thick paste comes together and then cook for 2 minutes until golden.

4. Stir in vegetable broth, bring it to a simmer, stir in black pepper and oregano, whisk well and cook for 15 minutes until gravy thickened to the desired level.

5. Add green beans, stir until mixed, remove the pan from heat, top beans with fried onions and bake for 15 minutes.

6. Serve straight away.

Nutrition: 191 Cal 10 g Fat 2 g Saturated Fat 22 g Carbohydrates 3.3 g Fiber 2.5 g Sugars 4.1 g Protein

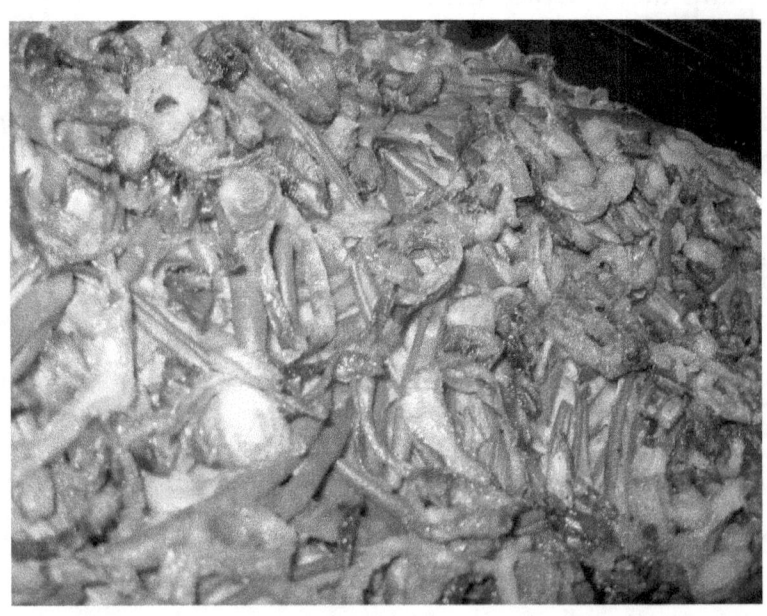

Pumpkin Risotto

Preparation Time: 5 minutes

Cooking Time: 20 minutes

Servings: 4

Ingredients:

1 cup Arborio rice

½ cup cooked and chopped pumpkin 1/2 cup mushrooms

1 rib of celery, diced

½ of a medium white onion, peeled, diced

½ teaspoon minced garlic

½ teaspoon salt

1/3 teaspoon ground black pepper 1 tablespoon olive oil

½ tablespoon coconut butter 1 cup pumpkin puree

2 cups vegetable stock

Directions:

1. Add oil on a saucepan, and when hot, add onion and celery, stir in garlic, and cook for 2 minutes

2. Add mushrooms, and cook for 5 minutes.

3.   Add rice, pour in pumpkin puree, then gradually pour in the stock until rice soaked up all the liquid and have turned soft.

4.   Add butter, remove the pan from heat, stir until creamy mixture comes together, and then serve.

Nutrition: 218.5 Cal 5.2 g Fat 1.5 g Saturated Fat 32.3 g Carbohydrates 1.3 g Fiber 3.8 g Sugars 6.3 g Protein;

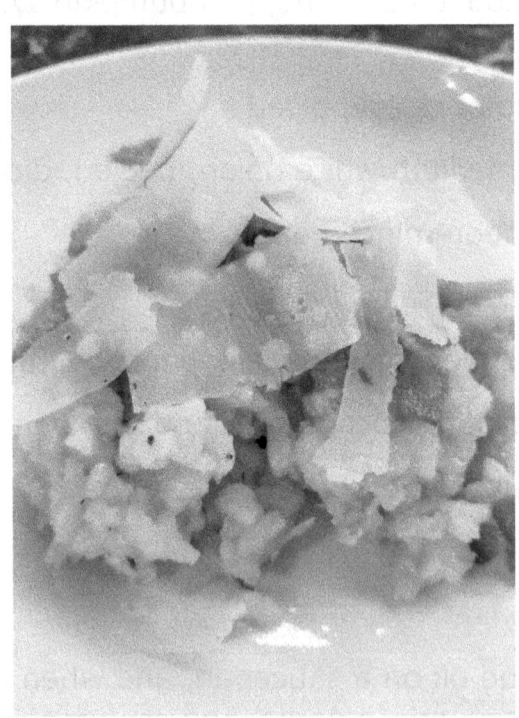

Brown Rice and Vegetable Stir-Fry

Preparation Time: 5 minutes

Cooking Time: 50 minutes

Servings: 4

Ingredients:

16-ounce tofu, extra-firm, pressed, drained, cut into ½-inch cubes

1 cup of brown rice

1 cup frozen broccoli florets

1 bell pepper, diced

1 white onion, peeled, diced

1 tablespoon minced garlic

½ teaspoon salt

1/3 teaspoon ground black pepper 1 tablespoon olive oil

2 cups vegetable broth

Directions:

1. Take a medium pot, place it over high heat, add brown rice, pour in vegetable broth, and bring it to a boil.

2. Switch heat to medium-low level, cover the pot with the lid and cook for 40 minutes, and when done, remove the pot and set aside until required.

3. Add oil to a skillet pot and when hot, add tofu pieces, onion, broccoli, and bell pepper, season with salt and black pepper, and cook for 5 minutes until sauté.

4. Add cooked rice, stir until mixed and continue cooking for 5 minutes.

5. Serve straight away.

Nutrition: 281.9 Cal 11.7 g Fat 1.7 g Saturated Fat 31.1 g Carbohydrates 9.7 g Fiber 2.1 g Sugars 20.1 g Protein;

Spicy Sesame & Edamame Noodles

Servings: 2

Ingredients

100 g Blue Dragon Whole-wheat Noodles 100 g vegetable 'noodles'

2 tsp coconut oil

2 shallots, sliced

2 tsp garlic

2 tsp ginger puree 1 red chili, sliced

3 tbsp. sesame seeds

100 g edamame beans, podded 2 tbsp. sesame oil

2 tbsp. Blue Dragon soy sauce

1 lime

Directions:

1. Boil the noodles, and set aside. Cook the vegetable noodles according to the guidelines and add the rest of the noodles.

2. Put oil on a pan and add garlic, ginger, and pepper. Cook for 2 minutes, and then add sesame seeds and bean sprouts. Cook for another 2 minutes, stir and stir to make sure nothing sticks to the bottom of the pot.

3.   Pour the noodles and the noodles into the pan and cook for 2 minutes.

4.   Turn off the heat and then add sesame oil, soy sauce, lemon juice, and mix. Serve with scattered coriander.

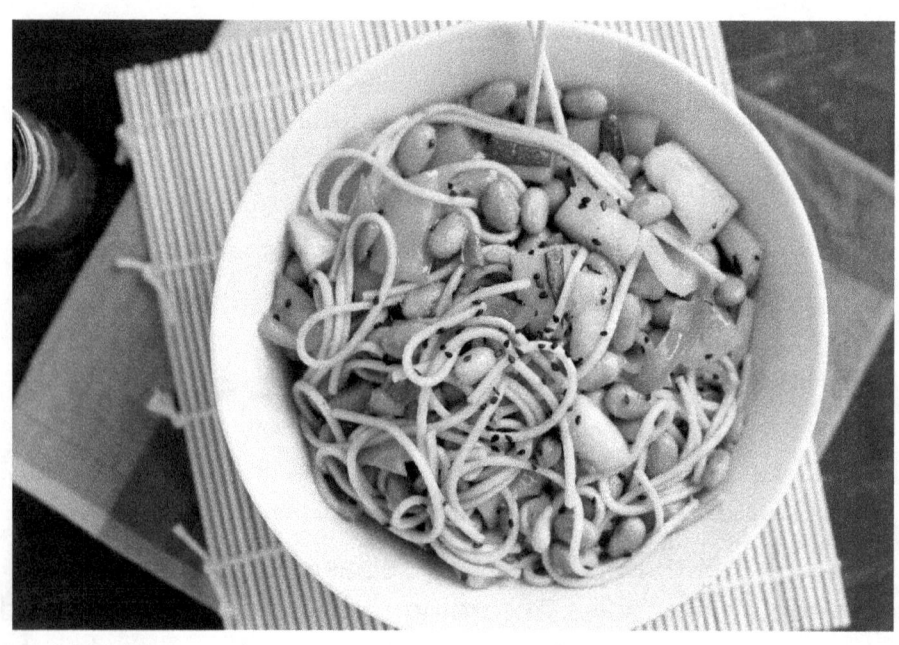

Quick & Easy Tomato and Herb Gigantes Beans

Servings: 2

Ingredients

2 tbsp. olive oil 1 onion

1 carrot

1 tsp ready-chopped garlic Protein content per serving garlic purée 1 Protein content per serving2 tsp paprika

400 g tin butterbeans

400 g tin chopped tomatoes 2 tbsp. tomato purée

1	tsp sugar

2	tsp dried oregano handful baby spinach handful fresh parsley 8-10 fresh mint leaves

Directions:

1. Chop onions and carrots, chop them finely, and add them to the bowl with garlic and paprika. Cook over medium heat for 2 minutes.

2.	Rinse and wash the potatoes and add to the pot, then add the greased tomatoes. Fill the empty tomato can in half with water and add it to the bowl with tomato puree, sugar, and oregano. Season well with salt and black pepper, boil, reduce at dawn, cover, and cook for 12-14 minutes.

3.	Chop the baby spinach approximately, then add them to the pot and cook for 2 minutes. Chop the parsley and mint almost and stir just before serving. Taste and adjust the seasoning if necessary, then serve with crusty bread and crispy green salad.

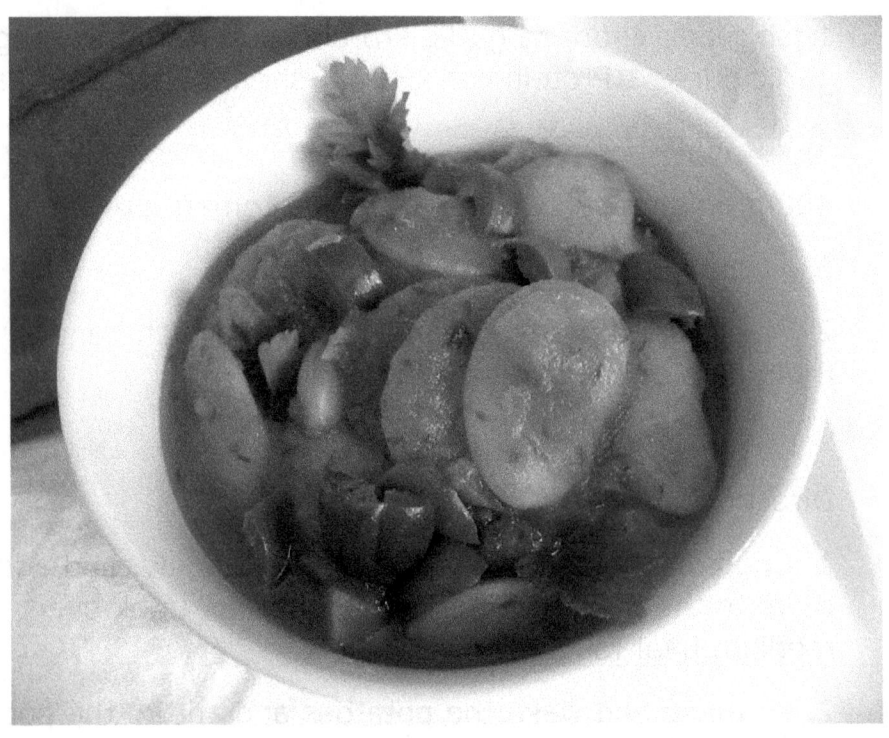

Creamy Vegan Spinach Pasta

Preparation Time: 20 minutes

Cooking Time: 5 minutes

Servings: 4

Ingredients:

2 cup cashews, soaked in water for 8 hours 2 tablespoons lemon juice

1   tablespoon olive oil 1½ cups vegetable broth

2   tablespoons fresh dill, chopped Red pepper flakes, to taste

10 oz. dried fusilli

½ cup almond milk, unflavored and unsweetened 2 tablespoons white miso paste

4 garlic cloves, divided

8-oz. fresh spinach, finely chopped

¼ cup scallions, chopped

Salt and black pepper, to taste

Directions:

1.   Make pasta.

2.   Cook as the package directions say and drain the pasta into a colander.

3. Dish out the pasta in a large serving bowl and add a dash of olive oil to prevent sticking.

4. Put the cashews, milk, miso, lemon juice, and 1 garlic clove into the food processor and blend until smooth.

5. Put oil in a pot. Add the remaining 3 cloves of garlic.

6. Sauté for about 1 minute and stir in the spinach and broth.

7. Raise the heat and simmer for about 4 minutes until the spinach is bright green and wilted.

8. Stir in the pasta and cashew mixture and season with salt and black pepper.

9. Top with scallions and dill and dish out into plates to serve.

Nutrition:

Calories: 94 Fat: 10g Protein: 8g Carbs: 17g Fiber: 6g

Vegan Bake Pasta with Bolognese Sauce and Cashew Cream

Preparation Time: 1 hour 10 minutes

Cooking Time: 20 minutes

Servings: 8

Ingredients:

For the Pasta:

1 packet penne pasta

For the Bolognese Sauce:

1 tablespoon soy sauce 1 small can lentils

1 tablespoon brown sugar

½ cup tomato paste

1	teaspoon garlic, crushed 1 tablespoon olive oil

2	tomatoes, chopped

1	onion, chopped

2	cups mushrooms, sliced Salt, to taste

Pepper, to taste

For the Cashew Cream:

1 cup raw cashews

½ lemon, squeezed

½ teaspoon salt

½ cup water

For the White Sauce:

1 teaspoon black pepper 1 teaspoon Dijon mustard

¼ cup nutritional yeast Sea salt, as required

2 cups coconut milk

3 tablespoons vegan butter

2 tablespoons all-purpose flour 1/3 cup vegetable broth

Directions:

1. Take a pot and boil water, add pasta to it, boil for 3 minutes, and set aside.

2. Fry onion and garlic, mushroom in olive oil, and add soy sauce to it.

3. Add sugar tomato paste, lentils, and canned tomato to it and let it simmer; Bolognese sauce is prepared.

4. Season it with salt and black pepper.

5. Add the lemon juice, cashews, water, and salt to the blender, blend for 2 minutes.

6. Add this to the sauce you have prepared and stir pasta in it.

7. Melt the vegan butter in a saucepan, add in the flour, and stir.

8. Add vegetable stock and coconut milk to it and whisk well.

9. Stir continuously and let it boil for about 5 minutes, then remove from heat.

10. Add Dijon mustard, nutritional yeast, black pepper, and sea salt.

11. Preheat the oven to 430°F.

12. Prepare a rectangular oven-safe dish by placing pasta and Bolognese sauce to it.

13. Pour the white sauce on it and bake for a time of 20-25 minutes.

Nutrition:

Calories: 314 Fat: 20g Protein: 21g Carbs: 15g Fiber: 6g

5 Ingredients Pasta

Preparation Time: 15 minutes

Cooking Time: 25 minutes

Servings: 5

Ingredients:

1 (25 oz.) jar marinara sauce Olive oil, as needed

1-pound dry vegan pasta

1 pound assorted vegetables, like red onion, zucchini, and tomatoes

¼ cup prepared hummus Salt, to taste

Directions:

1. Preheat the oven to 390°F and grease a large baking sheet.

2. Arrange the vegetables in a single layer on the baking sheet and sprinkle them with olive oil and salt.

3. Transfer into the oven and roast the vegetables for about 15 minutes.

4. Boil salted water in a large pot and cook the pasta according to the package directions.

5.   Drain the water when the pasta is tender and put the pasta in a colander.

6.   Mix the marinara sauce and hummus in a large pot to make a creamy sauce.

7.   Stir in the cooked vegetables and pasta to the sauce and toss to coat well.

8.   Dish out in a bowl and serve warm.

Nutrition: Calories: 415 Fat: 29g Protein: 33g Carbs: 5.5g Fiber: 2g

Sabich Sandwich

Preparation Time: 10 minutes

Cooking Time: 10 minutes

Servings: 4

Ingredients:

1/2 cup cooked white beans

2 medium potatoes, peeled, boiled, ½-inch thick sliced
1 medium eggplant, destemmed, ½-inch cubed

4 dill pickles, ¼-inch thick sliced

¼ teaspoon of sea salt 2 tablespoons olive oil

1/4 teaspoon harissa paste 1/2 cup hummus

1 tablespoon mayonnaise 4 pita bread pockets

1/2 cup tabbouleh salad

Directions:

1. Take a small frying pan, place it over medium-low heat, add oil and wait until it gets hot.

2. Season eggplant pieces with salt, add to the hot frying pan, and cook for 8 minutes until softened, and when done, remove the pan from heat.

3. Take a small bowl, place white beans in it, add harissa paste and mayonnaise and then stir until combined.

4. Assemble the sandwich and for this, place pita bread in a clean working space, smear generously with hummus, then cover half of each pita bread with potato slices and top with dill pickle slices.

5. Spoon 2 tablespoons of white bean mixture on each dill pickle, top with 3 tablespoons of cooked eggplant pieces and 2 tablespoons of tabbouleh salad, and then cover the filling with the other half of pita bread.

6. Serve straight away.

Nutrition: 386 Cal 13 g Fat 2 g Saturated Fat 56 g Carbohydrates 7 g Fiber 3 g Sugars 12 g Protein;

Tofu and Pesto Sandwich

Preparation Time: 10 minutes

Cooking Time: 15 minutes

Servings: 4

Ingredients:

2 blocks of tofu, firm, pressed, drained 8 slices of tomato

8 leaves of lettuce

1 ½ teaspoon dried oregano

½ cup green pesto

2 tablespoons olive oil

8 slices of sandwich bread

Directions:

1. Set the oven to 360 degrees F and let it preheat.

2. Cut tofu into thick slices, place them in a baking sheet, drizzle with oil and sprinkle with oregano, and bake the tofu pieces for 15 minutes until roasted.

3. Assemble the sandwich and for this, spread pesto on one side of each bread slice, then top four slices with

lettuce, tomato slices, and roasted tofu, and then cover with the other four slices.

4.   Serve straight away.

Nutrition: 277 Cal 9.1 g Fat 1.5 g Saturated Fat 33.1 g Carbohydrates 3.6 g Fiber 12.7 g Sugars 16.1 g Protein

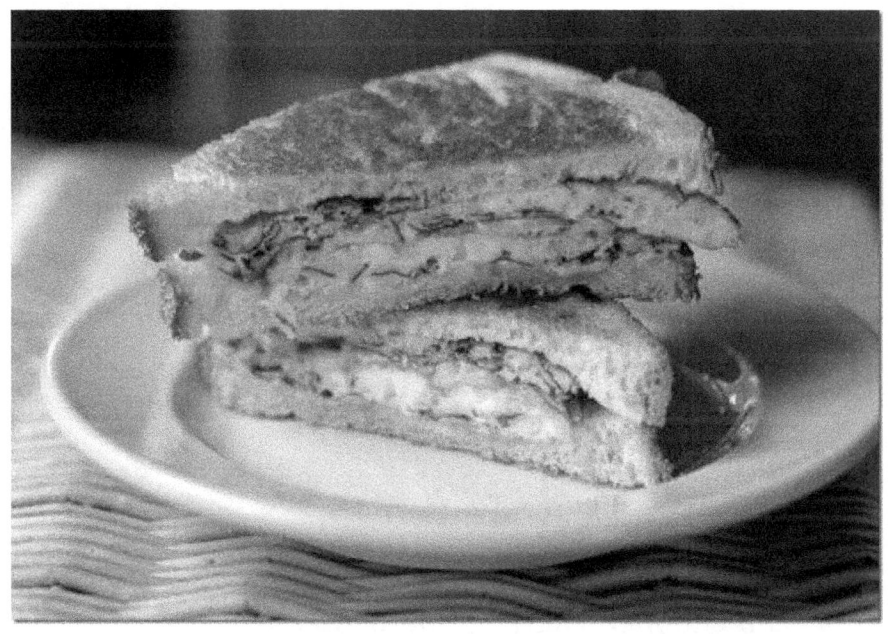

Chickpea and Mayonnaise Salad Sandwich

Preparation Time: 10 minutes

Cooking Time: 0 minutes

Servings: 4

Ingredients:

For the mayonnaise:

1/3 cup cashew nuts, soaked in boiling water for 10 minutes

½ teaspoon ground black pepper 1 teaspoon salt

6 teaspoons apple cider vinegar 2 teaspoon maple syrup

1/2 teaspoon Dijon mustard For the chickpea salad:

1 small bunch of chives, chopped 1 ½ cup sweetcorn

3 cups cooked chickpeas

To serve:

4 sandwich bread 4 leaves of lettuce

½ cup chopped cherry tomatoes

Directions:

1. Prepare the mayonnaise and for this, place all of its ingredients in a food processor and then pulse for 2

minutes until smooth, scraping the sides of the container frequently.

2. Take a medium bowl, place chickpeas in it, and then mash by using a fork until broken.

3. Add chives and corn, stir until mixed, then add mayonnaise and stir until well combined.

4. Assemble the sandwich and for this, stuff sandwich bread with chickpea salad, top each sandwich with a lettuce leaf and ¼ cup of chopped tomatoes and then serve.

Nutrition: 387 Cal 19 g Fat 5 g Saturated Fat 39.7 g Carbohydrates 7.2 g Fiber 4.9 g Sugars 10 g Protein

Tahini Broccoli

Preparation Time: 5 Minutes

Cooking Time: 15 Minutes

Servings: 4

Ingredients:

Toasted sesame seeds (.25 c.) Minced green onions Broccoli slaw (1 bag)

Soy sauce (2 teaspoons.) Sesame oil (1 Tablespoon.) Rice vinegar (1 Tablespoon.) White miso (2 Tablespoon.) Tahini (.25 c.)

Directions:

1. Take out a bowl and whisk together the soy sauce, oil, vinegar, miso, and tahini.
2. Add in the sesame seeds, green onions, and broccoli slaw. Set aside for 20 minutes and then serve.

Nutrition: Calories: 135 Carbs: 37g Fat: 0g Protein: 23g

Steamed Cauliflower

Preparation Time: 5 Minutes

Cooking Time: 15 Minutes

Servings: 4

Ingredients:

Red pepper flakes (1 teaspoon.) Salt (.5 teaspoon.)

Water (1 c.)

Cauliflower (1 head)

Directions:

1. Take the leaves off the cauliflower and then slice into florets.

2. Bring out a pan and bring some water to a boil. Add the steamer basket over it, and then add in the salt and florets.

3. Cover and let this steam for a bit. After five minutes, this should be nice and tender.

4. In a bowl, toss this with the red pepper flakes, and then serve.

Nutrition: Calories: 35 Carbs: 7g Fat: 0g Protein: 3g

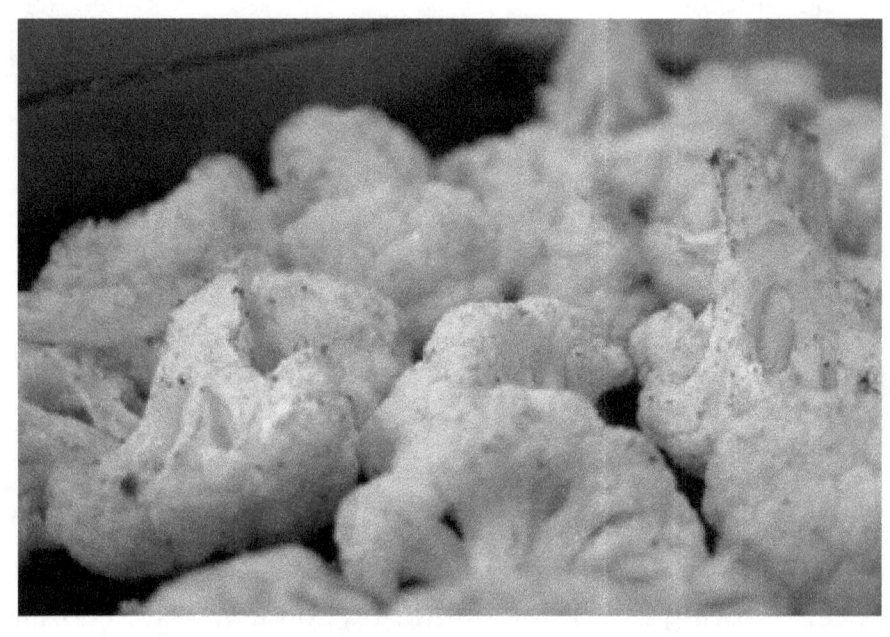

Cauliflower Tacos

Preparation Time: 10 Minutes

Cooking Time: 30 Minutes

Servings: 8

Ingredients:

For the roasted cauliflower

Chili powder (1 teaspoon.) Smoked paprika (2 teaspoons.) Nutritional yeast (2 Tablespoon.) Flour (2 Tablespoons.)

Olive oil (1 Tablespoon.) Cauliflower (1 head)

For the tacos

Lime wedges (Corn tortillas (8)

Guacamole (.5 c.) Mango salsa (.5 c.) Grated carrots (

Quartered cherry tomatoes (2 c.) Shredded lettuce (2 c.)

Directions:

1. Let the oven heat up to 340 degrees. Prepare a baking tray and set it to the side.

2. Toss the cauliflower with the oil and, in another bowl, mix all of the seasonings before adding it to the cauliflower.

3. Spread this onto the baking tray and add to the oven. After 20 minutes, this will be done, and you can take it out of the oven.

4. When the cauliflower is cooked, you can use those and the rest of the Ingredients: to assemble the tacos.

Nutrition: Calories: 198 Carbs: 32g Fat: 6g Protein: 7g

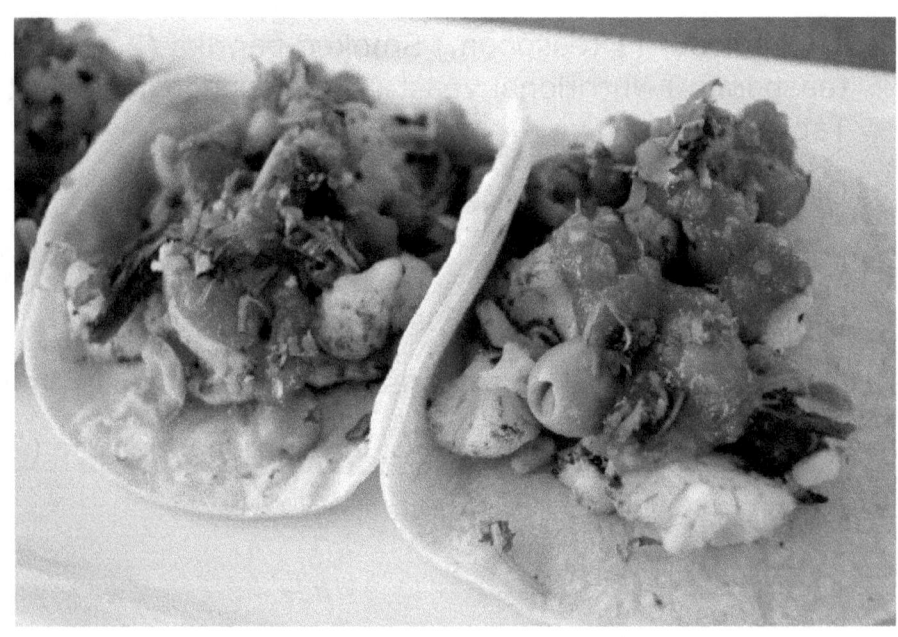

Sweet Potatoes

Preparation Time: 10 Minutes

Cooking Time: 35 Minutes

Servings: 4

Ingredients:

Salt (.5 teaspoon.)

Garlic powder (.5 teaspoon.) Dried thyme (.5 teaspoon.) Dried oregano (.5 teaspoon.) Smoked paprika (.5 teaspoon.) Cayenne pepper (.5 teaspoon.) Olive oil (2 teaspoons.)

Sweet potatoes (2 lbs.)

Directions:

1. Let the oven heat up to 400 degrees. Prepare a baking sheet with some parchment paper.
2. Wash the potatoes and then cube up. Move to a bowl and add the oil and potatoes together.
3. Combine the seasonings into another bowl and then sprinkle on top of the potatoes. Add this to the baking sheet and into the oven.
4. After 30 minutes of baking, take out of the oven and then serve warm.

Nutrition: Calories: 219 Carbs: 46g Fat: 3g Protein: 4g

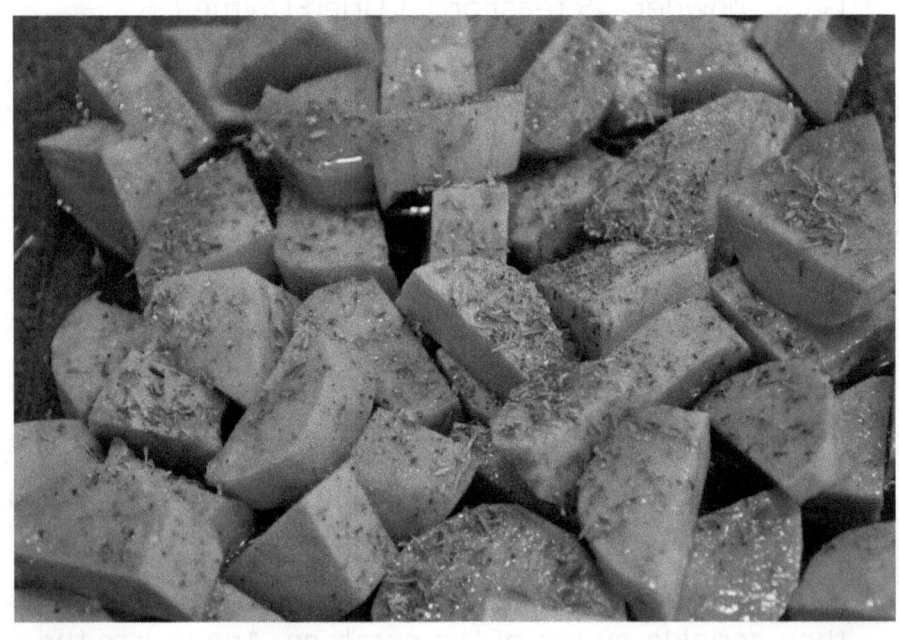

Smoky Meal

Preparation Time: 5 Minutes

Cooking Time: 10 Minutes

Servings: 6

Ingredients:

Chipotle powder (.25 teaspoon.) Smoked paprika (.25 teaspoon.) Pepper (.25 teaspoon.)

Salt (.5 teaspoon.)

Plain vegan yogurt (3 Tablespoons.) Rice vinegar (.25 c.)

Mayo (.33 c.)

Shredded cabbage (1 lb.)

Directions:

1. Bring out a big bowl and add the shredded cabbage inside. In another bowl, combine the chipotle powder, paprika, pepper, salt, sugar, yogurt, vinegar, and mayo.

2. Pour this over the cabbage and then mix it all up. Divide up and serve.

Nutrition: Calories: 73 Carbs: 8g Protein: 1g Fat: 4g

Roasted Vegetables and Quinoa Bowls

Preparation Time: 10 minutes

Cooking Time: 20 minutes

Servings: 4

Ingredients:

3 cups cooked quinoa For the Broccoli:

2 teaspoons minced garlic 4 cups broccoli florets

½ teaspoon salt

¼ teaspoon ground black pepper 4 teaspoons olive oil

For the Chickpeas:

4 teaspoons sriracha

3 cups cooked chickpeas 2 teaspoons olive oil

4 teaspoons soy sauce For the Roasted Sweet Potatoes:

2 teaspoons curry powder

2 small sweet potatoes, peeled, ¼-inch thick sliced 1/8 teaspoon salt

2 teaspoons sriracha 2 teaspoons olive oil

For the Chili-Lime Kale:

1/2 of a lime, juiced 4 cups chopped kale 1/8 teaspoon salt

1/8 teaspoon ground black pepper 1 teaspoon red chili powder

2 teaspoons olive oil

Directions:

1. Set the oven to 335 degrees F and let it preheat.

2. Prepare broccoli florets and for this, take a large bowl, place all of its ingredients in it, toss until well coated, then take a baking sheet lined with parchment paper and spread florets in a one- third portion of the sheet in a row.

3. Add chickpeas into the bowl, add their remaining ingredients, toss until well mixed, and spread them onto the baking sheet next to the broccoli florets.

4. Add sweet potatoes into the bowl, add their remaining ingredients, toss until well mixed, and spread them onto the baking sheet next to the chickpeas.

5. Place the baking sheet containing vegetables and chickpeas into the oven and then bake for 20 minutes until vegetables have turned tender and chickpeas are slightly crispy, turning halfway.

6. Meanwhile, prepare the kale and take a large skillet pan, place it over medium heat, add 1 teaspoon oil and when hot, add kale and cook for 5 minutes until tender.

7. Then season kale with salt, black pepper, and red chili powder, toss until mixed, and continue cooking for 3 minutes, set aside until required.

8. Assemble the bowl and for this, distribute quinoa evenly among four bowls, top evenly with broccoli, chickpeas, sweet potatoes, and kale and then serve.

Nutrition: 415 Cal 17 g Fat 2 g Saturated Fat 54 g Carbohydrates 8 g Fiber 5 g Sugars 16 g Protein;

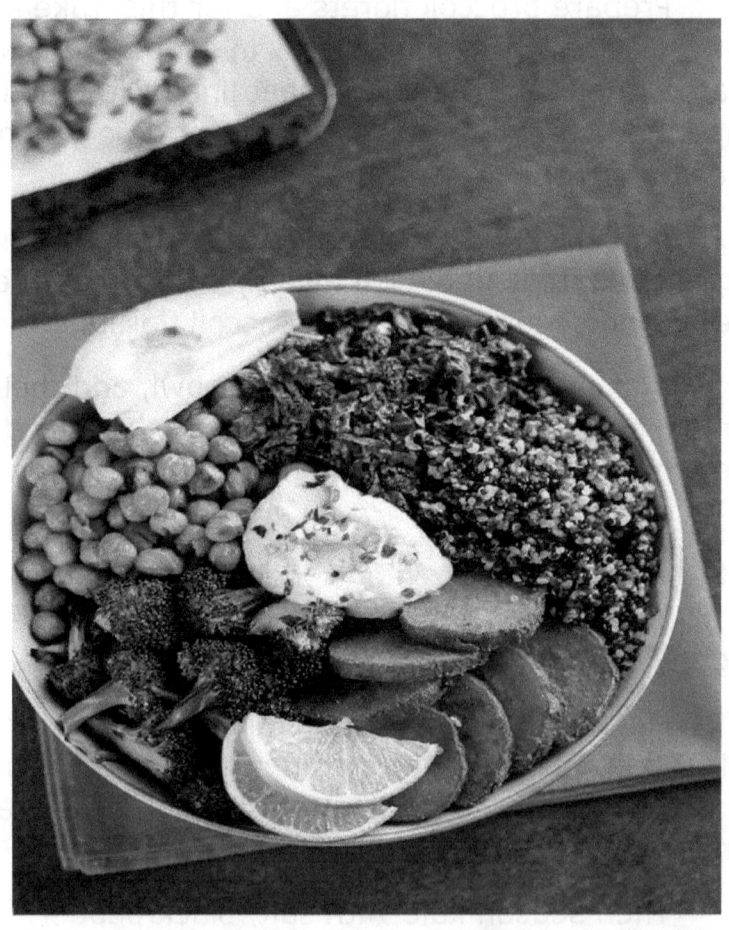

Sweet Potato and Quinoa Bowl

Preparation Time: 5 minutes

Cooking Time: 20 minutes

Servings: 4

Ingredients:

2 cups quinoa

1	cup diced red onion

2	cups diced sweet potato 1 1/2 cup raisins

1 cup sunflower seeds, shelled, unsalted 2 cups vegetable broth

Directions:

1.	Take a medium pot, place it over high heat, add quinoa, and sweet potatoes, pour in vegetable broth, stir until mixed and bring it to a boil.

2.	Then switch heat to medium-low level, cover pot with the lid, and cook for 20 minutes until the quinoa has cooked.

3.	When done, remove the pot from heat and fluff quinoa by using a fork.

4.	Add onion, raisins, and sunflower seeds, stir until mixed and transfer into a large bowl.

5.   Let it chill in the refrigerator for 30 minutes and then serve.

Nutrition: 204 Cal 7 g Fat 3 g Saturated Fat 31 g Carbohydrates 3 g Fiber 11 g Sugars 3 g Protein

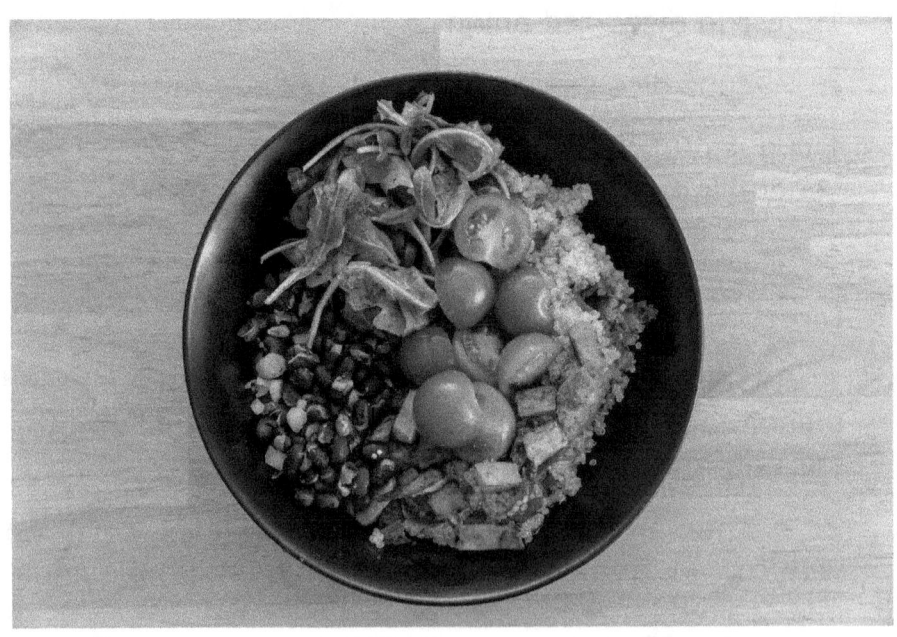

Chickpea Salad Bites

Preparation Time: 15 minutes

Cooking Time: 0 minutes

Servings: 4

Ingredients:

For the Bread:

2 tablespoons chopped parsley 1 small green chili pepper

1/3 cup of raisins

1	teaspoon garlic powder

½ teaspoon salt

1/3 teaspoon ground black pepper

½ teaspoon smoked paprika

½ tablespoon maple syrup

½ teaspoon cayenne pepper

2	tablespoons balsamic vinegar

1	1/2 cups crumbled rye bread, whole-grain For the Salad:

2	scallions, chopped

1/3 cup chopped pickles

2 tablespoons chopped chives and more for topping

½ teaspoon minced garlic 1 ½ cup cooked chickpeas 1 lemon, juiced

½ teaspoon salt

¼ tsp pepper 1 tablespoon poppy seeds

1 teaspoon mustard paste 1/3 cup coconut yogurt

Directions:

1.	Prepare the bread, and for this, place all of its ingredients in a food processor and then pulse for 1 minute until just combined; don't overmix.

2.	Then make bites of the bread mixture, and for this, take a 2.3- inch round cookie cutter, add 2 tablespoons of the bread mixture, press it into the cutter, and gently lift it out; repeat with the remaining batter to make seven more bites.

3.	Prepare the salad and for this, take a large bowl, add chickpeas in it, then add chives, scallion, pickles, and garlic, and then mash chickpeas by using a fork until broken.

4.	Add remaining ingredients for the salad and stir until well mixed.

5.	Assemble the bites and for this, top each prepared bread bite generously with prepared salad, sprinkle with chives and poppy seeds, and then serve.

Nutrition: 210 Cal 4 g Fat 1 g Saturated Fat 36 g Carbohydrates 6 g Fiber 4 g Sugars 7 g Protein;

Avocado and Chickpeas Lettuce Cups

Preparation Time: 10 minutes

Cooking Time: 0 minutes

Servings: 4

Ingredients:

2 small avocados, peeled, pitted, diced 8 ounces hearts of palm

¾ cup cooked chickpeas 1/2 cup cucumber, diced

1 tablespoon minced shallots 2 cups mixed greens

1 tablespoon Dijon mustard 1 lime, zested, juiced

2 tablespoons chopped cilantro and more for topping 2/3 teaspoon salt

1/3 teaspoon ground black pepper 1 tablespoon apple cider vinegar 2 ½ tablespoons olive oil

Directions:

1. Take a medium bowl, add shallots and cilantro in it, stir in salt, black pepper, mustard, vinegar, lime juice, and zest until just mixed, and then slowly mix in olive oil until combined.

2. Add cucumber, hearts of palm, and chickpeas, stir until mixed, fold in avocado and then top with some more cilantro.

3. Distribute mixed greens among four plates, top with chickpea mixture, and then serve.

Nutrition: 280 Cal 12.6 g Fat 1.5 g Saturated Fat 32.8 g Carbohydrates 9.3 g Fiber 1.2 g Sugars 7.6 g Protein;

Pappardelle with Cavolo Nero (cabbage) & Walnut Sauce

Servings: 2

Ingredients:

200 g Cavolo Nero (cabbage) 150 g walnut pieces

250 g Pappardelle pasta 1 slice bread

150 g dairy-free milk

2 tbsp. parsley

olive oil

Directions:

1.	Remove the kale stems and cut them into slices of protein per serving.

2.	Heat a pan, peel the nuts (no oil needed), and bake over medium heat for 2-3 minutes. Turn off the heat and reserve.

3.	Soak Cavolo Nero for 1 minute, then use a slotted spoon or tweezers to remove it with a sieve or stain (remove the boiling water in the pot).

4.	Simmer pappardelle for 8-10 minutes.

5.	Meanwhile, sprinkle nuts, bread, milk protein content in each serving of milk, parsley, garlic, and

Parmesan (if used) in a blender or food mixer and mix until consistent. Reach the thick sauce, beat it — season well with salt and black pepper.

6. Heat the pan again, add a little olive oil, and put it in Kawlow, Norway. Cook for 3-4 minutes and turn off the heat.

7. Drain pasta and return it to the pot. Tilt and add the walnut sauce to combine. Finally, add cavolo Nero, overlay, and then divide between two dishes.

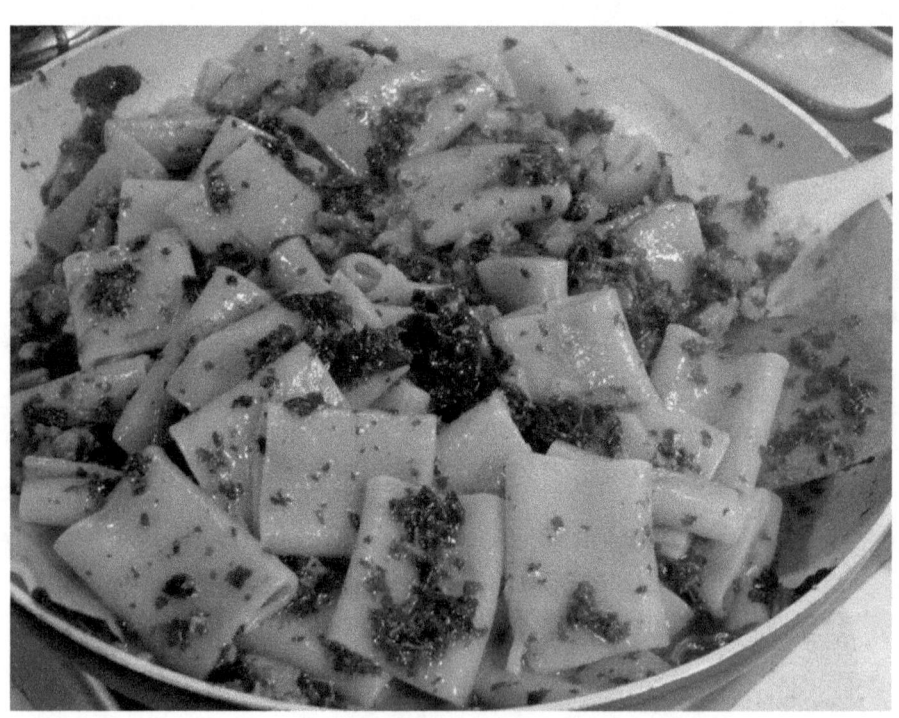

Veggie Sausage & Sun-Dried Tomato One Pot Pasta

Servings: 4

Ingredients:

2 tbsp. oil

3 sausages

1 onion, peeled and sliced 400 g pasta shells

200 g cherry tomatoes, halved

6-8 sun-dried tomatoes, roughly chopped

1-liter water

2 tsp powder

100 ml dairy-free cream (I used soya) 100 g fresh baby spinach

Instructions:

1. Fry the sausage and onion until the sausages brown. Carefully separate them from the pan, cut each piece into slices into 4 parts, and then return to the pot for another 2 minutes.

2. Add pasta, tomatoes, sun-dried tomatoes, water, and powder to the pot. Cook for 13 minutes, until the pasta is well cooked.

3.   Add to the pot the cream and spinach, then cook for another minute until the spinach has vanished.

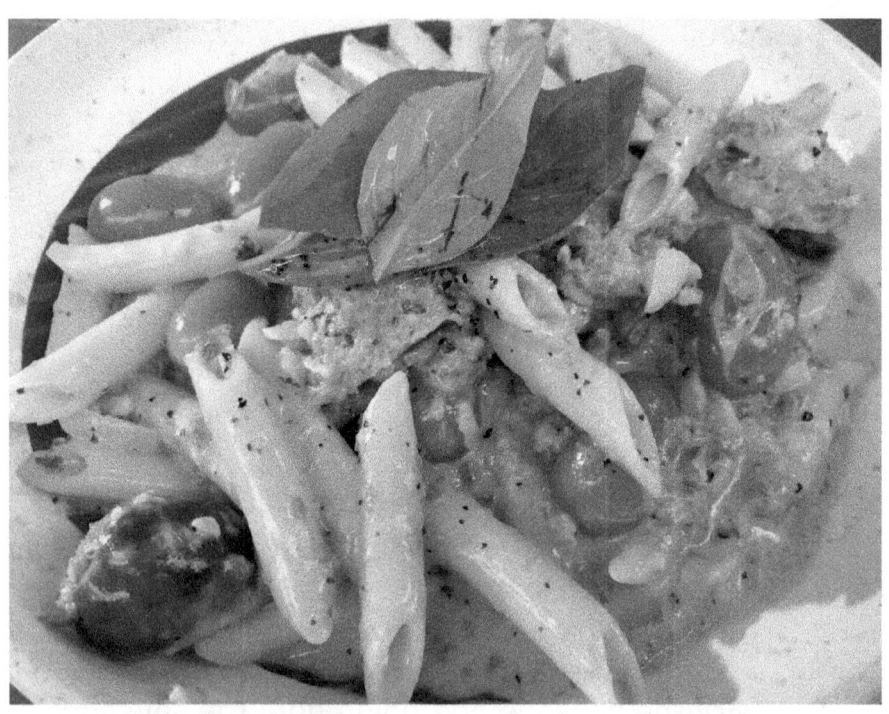

Chickpea Sunflower Sandwich

Preparation Time: 15 minutes

Cooking Time: 10 minutes

Servings: 2

Ingredients:

For The Sandwich:

One ¾ cup cooked chickpeas 1/4 cup chopped red onion

1/4 cup roasted sunflower seeds, unsalted

½ teaspoon salt

¼ teaspoon ground black pepper 1 tablespoon maple syrup

1/2 teaspoon Dijon mustard

3 tablespoons vegan mayonnaise 2 tablespoons fresh dill

4 pieces of rustic bread For The Garlic Herb Sauce:

1 teaspoon minced garlic 1/2 of lemon, juiced

½ teaspoon of sea salt 1 teaspoon dried dill

¼ dried dill

1/4 cup hummus

¼ cup almond milk, unsweetened For Topping:

1 avocado, pitted, sliced

1 medium white onion, peeled, sliced

½ cup chopped lettuce

1 medium tomato, sliced

Directions:

1.   Prepare the garlic herb sauce and for this, take a medium bowl, place and whisk all of its ingredients until combined, set aside until combined.

2.   Take a medium bowl, add chickpeas in it, and then mash by using a fork until broken.

3.   Then add onion, dill, sunflower seeds, salt, black pepper, mustard, maple syrup, and mayonnaise and stir until well combined.

4.   Place a medium skillet pan over medium heat, add bread slices, and cook for 3 minutes per side until toasted.

5.   Spread chickpea mixture on one side of two bread slices, top with prepared garlic herb sauce, avocado, onion, tomato, and lettuce, and cover with the other two slices.

6.   Serve straight away.

Nutrition: 532 Cal 30 g Fat 4 g Saturated Fat 52 g Carbohydrates 14 g Fiber

8 g Sugars 17 g Protein;

Stir Fry Noodles

Preparation Time: 10 minutes

Cooking Time: 8 minutes

Servings: 4

Ingredients:

1 cup broccoli,

1 cup red bell pepper,1 cup mushrooms, chopped

1 large onion, chopped

1 batch Stir Fry Sauce, prepared Salt and black pepper, to taste

2 cups spaghetti, cooked 4 garlic cloves, minced 2 tablespoons sesame oil

Directions:

1. Put oil in a pan. Add garlic, onions, bell pepper, broccoli, mushrooms.

2. Sauté for about 5 minutes and add spaghetti noodles and stir fry sauce.

3. Mix well and cook for 3 more minutes.

4. Dish out in plates and serve to enjoy.

Nutrition: Calories: 567 Fat: 48g Carbs: 6g Fiber: 4g Protein: 33g

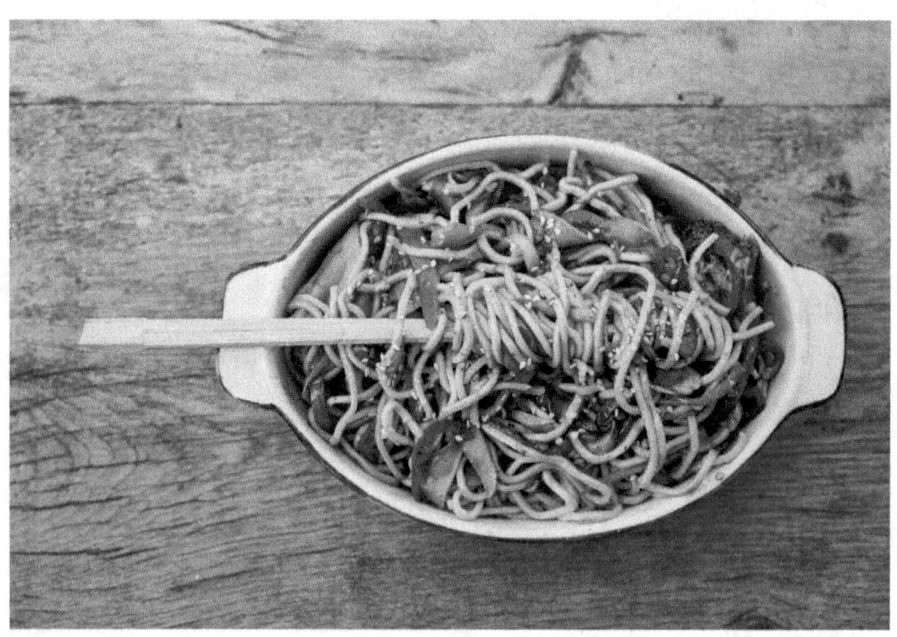

Spicy Sweet Chili Veggie Noodles

Preparation Time: 10 minutes

Cooking Time: 7 minutes

Servings: 2

Ingredients:

For Sauce:

2 head of broccoli

1 onion, finely sliced

1	tablespoon olive oil 1 courgette, halved

2	nests of whole-wheat noodles 5 oz. mushrooms, sliced

3	tablespoons soy sauce

¼ cup sweet chili sauce 1 teaspoon Sriracha

1	tablespoon peanut butter 2 tablespoons boiled water For Topping

2	teaspoons sesame seeds

2 teaspoons dried chili flakes

Directions:

1.	Put oil on medium heat in a saucepan and add onions.

2.   Sauté for about 2 minutes and add broccoli, courgette, and mushrooms.

3.   Cook for about 5 minutes, stirring occasionally.

4.   Whisk sweet chili sauce, soy sauce, Sriracha, water, and peanut butter in a bowl.

5.   Cook the noodles as the packet instructions say and add to the vegetables.

6.   Stir in the sauce and top with dried chili flakes and sesame seeds to serve.

Nutrition:

Calories: 351 Fat: 27g Protein: 25g Carbs: 2g Fiber: 1g

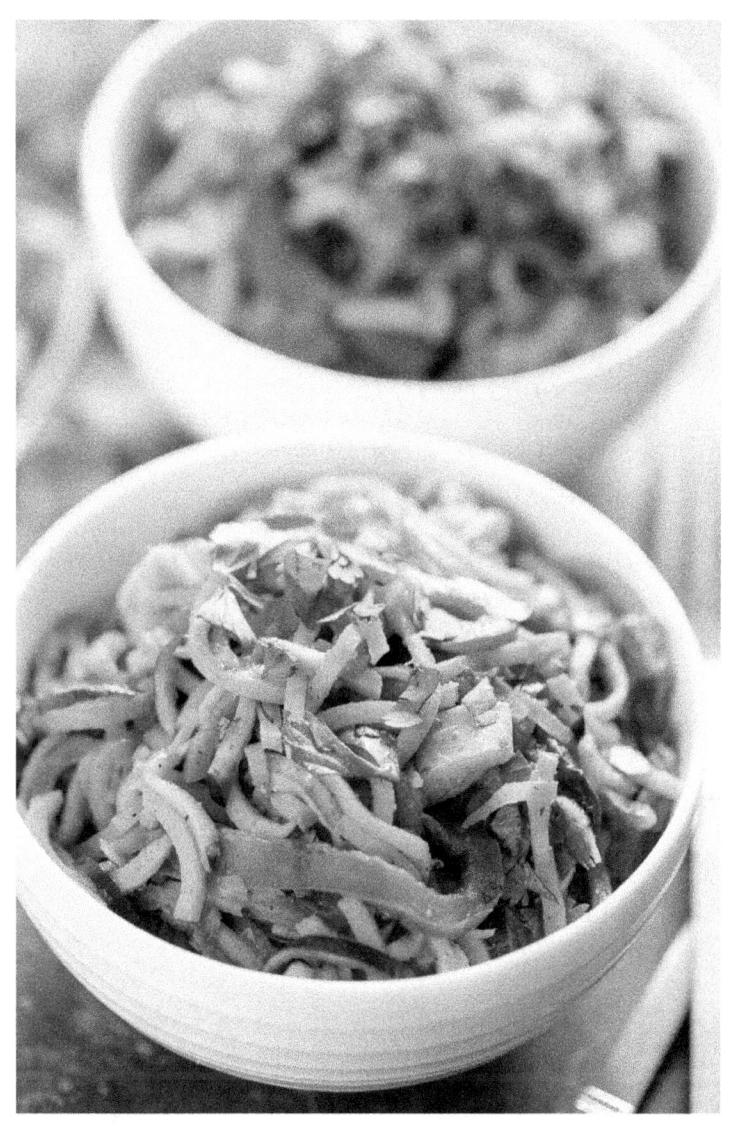

Creamy Vegan Mushroom Pasta

Preparation Time: 10 minutes

Cooking Time: 30 minutes

Servings: 6

Ingredients:

2   cups frozen peas, thawed

3   tablespoons flour, unbleached

3 cups almond breeze, unsweetened 1 tablespoon nutritional yeast

1/2 cup parsley, chopped, plus extra for garnish

¼ cup olive oil

1-pound pasta of choice 4 cloves garlic, minced 2/3 cup shallots, chopped

8 cups mixed mushrooms, sliced Salt, and black pepper, to taste

Directions:

1.   Take a bowl and boil pasta in salted water.

2.   Put olive oil in a pan.

3.   Add mushrooms, garlic, shallots, and ½ tsp salt and cook for 15 minutes.

4. Sprinkle flour on the vegetables and stir for a minute while cooking.

5. Add almond beverage; stir frequently.

6. Let it simmer for 5 minutes and add pepper to it.

7. Cook for 3 more minutes and remove from heat.

8. Stir in nutritional yeast.

9. Add peas, salt, and pepper.

10. Cook for another minute and add

11. Add pasta to this sauce.

12. Garnish and serve!

Nutrition: Calories: 364 Fat: 28g Protein: 24g Carbs: 24g

Fiber: 2g

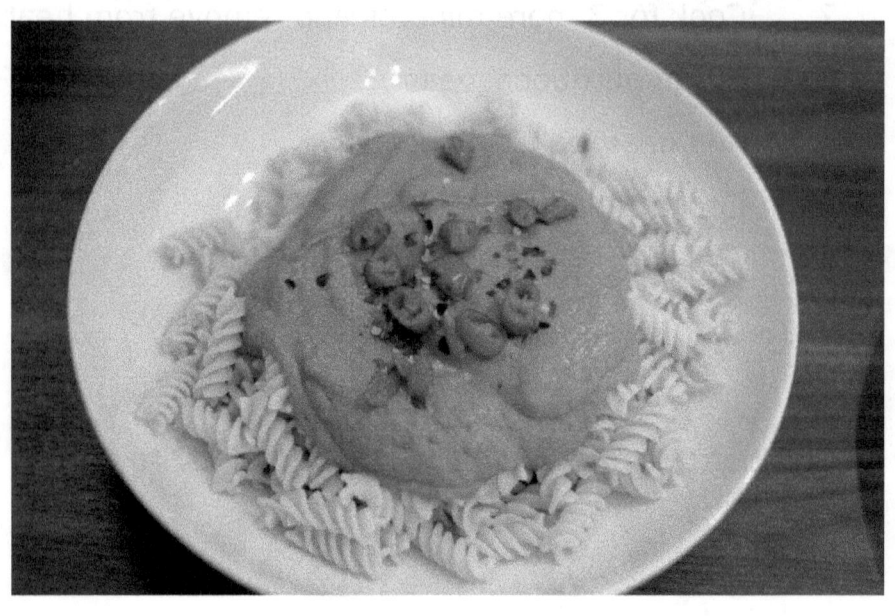

Vegan Chinese Noodles

Preparation Time: 15 minutes

Cooking Time: 8 minutes

Servings: 4

Ingredients:

10 oz. mixed oriental mushrooms, such as oyster, shiitake, and enoki, cleaned and sliced

7 oz. thin rice noodles, cooked as the packet instructions say and drained

2 garlic cloves, minced 1 fresh red chili

7 oz. courgettes, sliced

6 spring onions, reserving the green part 1 teaspoon cornflour

1	tbsp agave syrup 1 teaspoon sesame oil

100g baby spinach, chopped Hot chili sauce, to serve

2(1-inch) pieces of ginger

½ bunch fresh coriander, chopped 4 tablespoons vegetable oil

2	tablespoons low-salt soy sauce

½ tablespoon rice wine 2 limes, to serve

Directions:

1. Put oil and mushrooms in a pan.

2. Sauté for about 4 minutes and add garlic, chili, ginger, courgette, coriander stalks, and the white part of the spring onions.

3. Sauté for about 3 minutes until softened and lightly golden.

4. Meanwhile, combine the cornflour and 2 tablespoons of water in a bowl.

5. Add soy sauce, agave syrup, sesame oil, and rice wine to the cornflour mixture.

6. Put this mixture in the pan to the veggie mixture and cook for about 3 minutes until thickened.

7. Add the spinach and noodles and mix well.

8. Stir in the coriander leaves and top with lime wedges, hot chili sauce, and reserved spring onions to serve.

Nutrition:

Calories: 314 Fat: 22g Protein: 26g Carbs: 8g Fiber: 0.3g

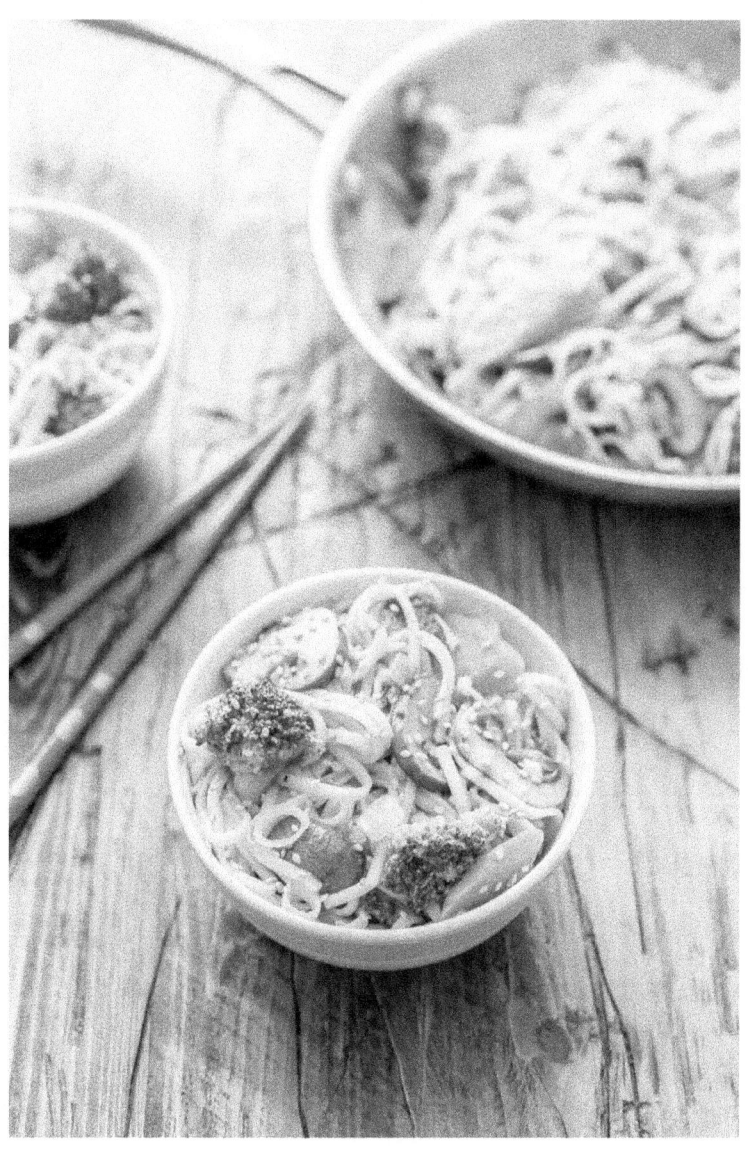

Vegetable Penne Pasta

Preparation Time: 15 minutes

Cooking Time: 20 minutes

Servings: 6

Ingredients:

½ large onion, chopped 2 celery sticks, chopped

½ tablespoon ginger paste

½ cup green bell pepper 1½ tablespoons soy sauce

½ teaspoon parsley

Salt and black pepper, to taste

½ pound penne pasta, cooked 2 large carrots, diced

½ small leek, chopped 1 tablespoon olive oil

½ teaspoon garlic paste

½ tablespoon Worcester sauce

½ teaspoon coriander 1 cup water

Directions:

1. Put oil in a wok on medium heat and add onions, garlic, and ginger paste.

2. Sauté for about 3 minutes and stir in all bell pepper, celery sticks, carrots, and leek.

3. Sauté for about 5 minutes and add remaining ingredients except for pasta.

4. Cover the lid and cook for about 12 minutes.

5. Stir in the cooked pasta and dish out to serve warm.

Nutrition:

Calories: 385 Fat: 29g Protein: 26g Carbs: 12g Fiber: 1g

Chestnut Mushroom Bourguignon

Servings: 2

Ingredients:

2 tbsp. olive oil

2 shallots or 1 small onion

10 baby Protein content per serving chantenay carrots

1 tsp ready-chopped garlic Protein content per serving garlic puree 250 g chestnut mushrooms

100 g button mushrooms l½ tbsp. plain flour

200 ml red wine

150 ml of boiling water

1 tsp vegetable stock powder 1 tbsp. tomato puree

handful fresh parsley

Directions:

1.   Heat the oil in a large skillet or large skillet over high heat. Chop the peels and mash, and add the garlic to the pot. Cut and halve carrot lengths (quadruple in large size) and add to the pan.

2.   Chop the brown mushrooms into four sections and clean the

Mushrooms. Cook for 2 and half minutes.

3. Stir the flour through the mushrooms, then add the red wine. Add water, powdered broth, and tomato puree. Cook over medium heat to form a thick and bright sauce, and the mushrooms are cooked inside but not too soft. Try and add black pepper, salt, and pepper if necessary.

4. Chop the parsley approximately and stir approximately two-thirds through the bourbon, then wash the plate and sprinkle with the remaining parsley.

Broad Bean, Fennel & Baby Carrot Pilaf
Servings: 2

Ingredients:

1 onion

1 fennel bulb

1 tsp garlic puree Protein content per serving garlic

2 tbsp oil

220 g broad beans

110 g carrots

200 g basmati rice

400 ml vegetable stock

1 lemon

40 g walnuts

handful fresh parsley

Directions:

1. Peel and chop the onions, chop the fennel and chop finely and chop the garlic cloves. Fry the onion and garlic for 1.5 minutes to soften.

2. Chop the baby carrots and cook in half. Add them to the pot with beans and basmati rice, then store the vegetables. Bring to a boil, sauté in a sauce and cook for 12 minutes or until the rice is cooked. At the end of

cooking, check the rice for a few minutes, and if it looks too dry, add a little more water.

3.   Meanwhile, chop the nuts and parsley leaves and sprinkle them with lemon. When the rice is cooked, pour the lemon juice and crush the nuts and parsley. Serve immediately if necessary.

Spelled Spaghetti with Avocado Pesto

Servings: 2

Ingredients:

200 g spelled spaghetti (white or whole-wheat)

13 asparagus spears, sliced

100 g peas

1 and half avocado

78 g nuts

1 garlic, peeled and crushed zest

juice of 1 lemon

2 tbsp. extra virgin olive oil 50 g fresh basil

salt

Directions:

1. Bring a large pot of boiling water and add spaghetti. After 5 minutes of cooking (or 8 boxes of whole spaghetti), add the peas and asparagus and cook for 2-3 minutes until the pasta is cooked and the asparagus is cooked naturally.

2. While preparing the spaghetti, place all remaining ingredients in the blender or meal and cook for a minute. Add 2-3 tablespoons of water and stain again, and add a little water once to achieve a thick sauce. Try and add more salt if necessary.

3. Drain the spaghetti, return them to the pot, and then stir over the sauce over low heat to cool.

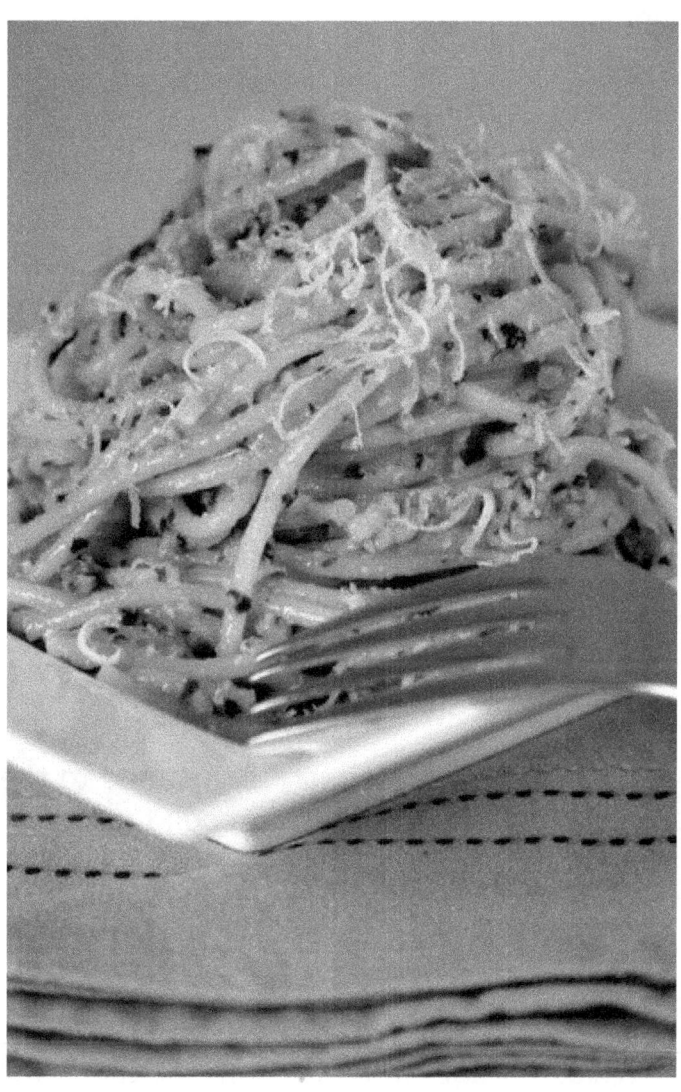

Mushrooms Sandwich

Preparation Time: 10 minutes

Cooking Time: 5 minutes

Servings: 4

Ingredients:

8 cherry tomatoes, halved 2 ounces of baby spinach

20 ounces of oyster mushrooms 2/3 teaspoon salt

1/3 teaspoon ground black pepper 2 tablespoons olive oil

4 tablespoons of barbecue sauce 8 slices of bread, toasted

Directions:

1. Place a griddle pan over medium-high heat, grease it with oil and let it preheat.

2. Cut mushroom into thin strips, add to the hot griddle pan, drizzle with oil and cook for 5 minutes until done.

3. Transfer grilled mushrooms into a medium bowl, season with salt and black pepper, add barbecue sauce and toss until mixed.

4. Spread prepared mushroom mixture evenly on four bread slices, top with spinach and cherry tomatoes, then cover with the other four slices and serve.

Nutrition: 350 Cal 11 g Fat 3 g Saturated Fat 46 g Carbohydrates 9 g Fiber

7.2 g Sugars 12.1 g Protein;

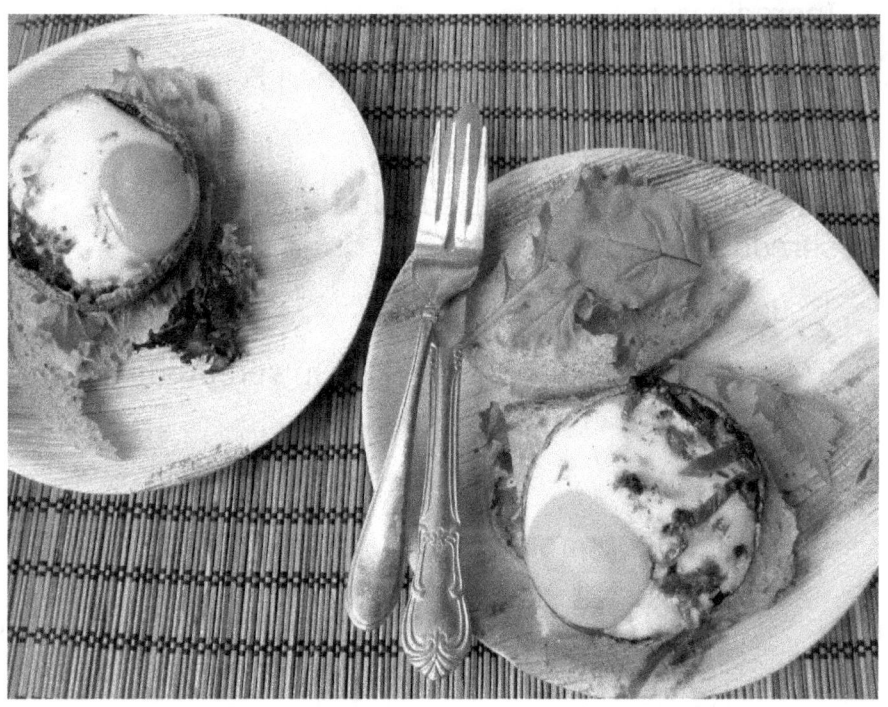

Rainbow Taco Boats

Preparation Time: 10 minutes

Cooking Time: 0 minutes

Servings: 4

Ingredients:

1 head romaine lettuce, destemmed For the Filling:

1/2 cup alfalfa sprouts

1 medium avocado, peeled, pitted, cubed 1 cup shredded carrots

1 cup cherry tomatoes

3/4 cup sliced red cabbage 1/2 cup sprouted hummus dip 1 tablespoon hemp seeds

For the Sauce:

1 tablespoon maple syrup 1/3 cup tahini

1/8 teaspoon sea salt

2 tablespoons lemon juice 3 tablespoons water

Directions:

1. Take a medium bowl, add all the ingredients in it and whisk until well combined.

2. Assemble the boats and for this, arrange lettuce leaves in twelve portions, top each with hummus, and the remaining ingredients for the filling.

3. Serve with prepared sauce.

Nutrition: 314 Cal 23.6 g Fat 4 g Saturated Fat 23.2 g Carbohydrates 9.3 g Fiber 6.2 g Sugars 8 g Protein

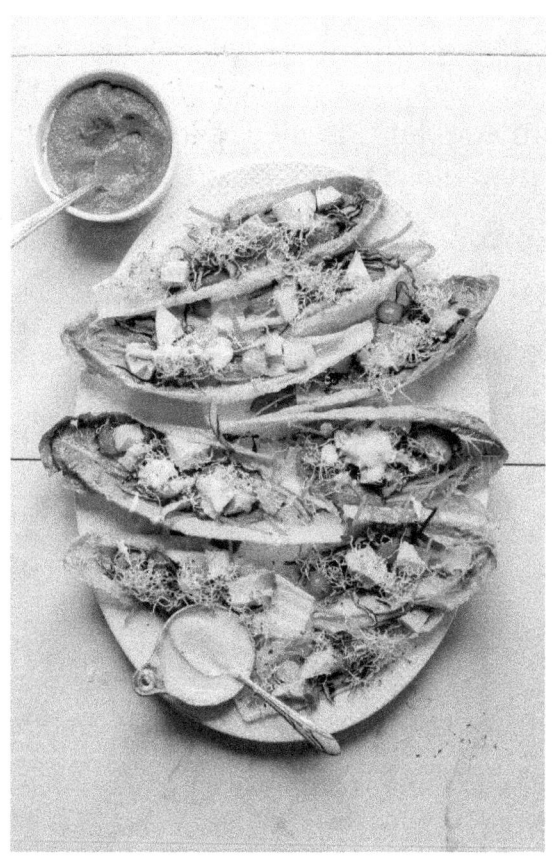

Eggplant Sandwich

Preparation Time: 10 minutes

Cooking Time: 25 minutes

Servings: 4

Ingredients:

For the Sandwich:

2 ciabatta buns

1 medium eggplant, peeled, sliced, soaked in salted water 1 medium tomato, sliced

1/2 of a medium cucumber, sliced 1/2 cup arugula

4 tablespoons mayo For the Marinade:

1 teaspoon agave syrup 1/4 teaspoon salt

1/4 teaspoon ground black pepper 1 teaspoon smoked paprika

1 tablespoon soy sauce 1 tablespoon olive oil

Directions:

1. Set the oven to 350 degrees F and let it preheat.

2. Place the ingredients in it and whisk until combined.

3. Drain the eggplant slices, pat dry with a kitchen towel, brush with prepared marinade, arrange them on a baking sheet and then bake for 20 minutes until done.

4. Assemble the sandwich, and for this, slice the bread in half lengthwise, top with baked eggplant slices, tomato, cucumber slices, and sprinkle with salt and black pepper.

5. Top with arugula leaves, cover with the top half of the bun, and then cover aluminum foil.

6. Preheat the grill over a medium-high heat setting, and when hot, place prepared sandwiches and grill for 3 to 5 minutes until toasted.

7. Cut each sandwich through the foil into half and serve.

Nutrition: 688 Cal 15 g Fat 2 g Saturated Fat 118 g Carbohydrates 7 g Fiber

7 g Sugars 21 g Protein;

Lentil, Cauliflower and Grape Salad

Preparation Time: 10 minutes

Cooking Time: 25 minutes

Servings: 4

Ingredients:

For the Cauliflower:

1 medium head of cauliflower, cut into florets 1/4 teaspoon sea salt

1 1/2 tablespoons curry powder

1 1/2 tablespoons melted coconut oil For the Tahini Dressing:

2 tablespoons tahini 1/8 teaspoon salt

1.8 teaspoon ground black pepper 4 1/2 tablespoons green curry paste

1 tablespoon maple syrup 2 tablespoons lemon juice 2 tablespoons water

For the Salad:

1 cup cooked lentils

4 tablespoons chopped cilantro 1 cup red grapes, halved

6 cups mixed greens

Directions:

1. Set the oven it to 400 degrees F and let it preheat.

2. Prepare the cauliflower and for this, take a medium bowl, place cauliflower florets in it, drizzle with oil, season with salt and curry powder, toss until mixed.

3. Take a baking sheet, line it with a parchment sheet, spread cauliflower florets in it, and then bake for 25 minutes until tender and nicely golden brown.

4. Meanwhile, prepare the tahini dressing, and for this, take a medium bowl, whisk the ingredients until combined, set aside until required.

5. Assemble the salad and for this, take a large salad bowl, add roasted cauliflower florets, lentils, grapes, and mixed greens, drizzle with prepared tahini dressing and toss until well combined.

6. Serve straight away.

Nutrition: 420 Cal 14 g Fat 5 g Saturated Fat 37.6 g Carbohydrates 9.8 g Fiber 12.8 g Sugars 10.8 g Protein;

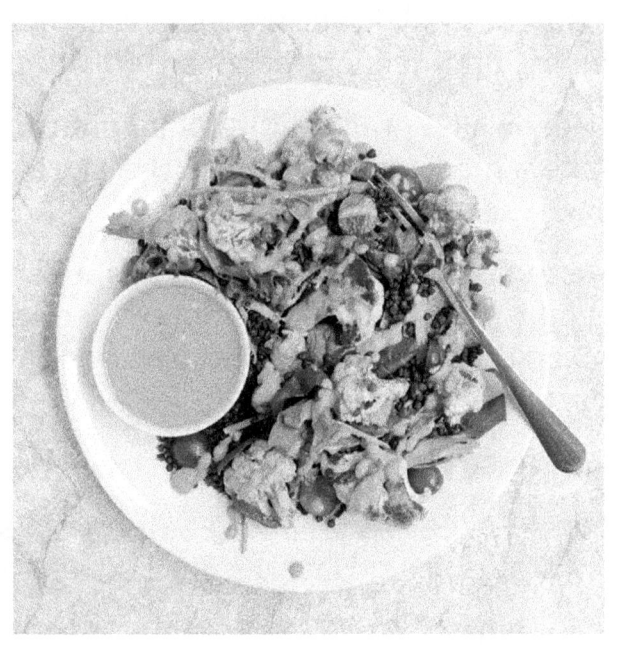

Spaghetti in Spicy Tomato Sauce

Preparation Time: 15 minutes

Cooking Time: 40 minutes

Servings: 4

Ingredients:

1 pound dried spaghetti 1 red bell pepper, diced 4 garlic cloves, minced

1 teaspoon red pepper flakes, crushed 2 (14-oz.) cans diced tomatoes

1	(6-oz.) can tomato paste

2	teaspoons vegan sugar, granulated 2 tablespoons olive oil

1 medium onion, diced 1 cup dry red wine

1 teaspoon dried thyme

½ teaspoon fennel seed, crushed 1½ cups coconut milk, full-fat Salt, and black pepper, to taste

Directions:

1.	Make pasta.

2.	Cook as the package directions say and drain the pasta into a

Colander.

3. Dish out the pasta in a large serving bowl and add a dash of olive oil to prevent sticking.

4. Heat 2 tbsp of olive oil over medium heat in a large pot and add garlic, onion, and bell pepper.

5. Sauté for about 5 minutes and stir in the wine, thyme, fennel, and red pepper flakes.

6. Allow simmering on high heat for about 5 minutes until the liquid is reduced by about half.

7. Add diced tomatoes and tomato paste and allow to simmer for about 20 minutes, stirring occasionally.

8. Mix milk and sugar and simmer for about 10 more minutes.

9. Season with salt and black pepper and pour the sauce over the pasta.

10. Toss to coat well and dish out in plates to serve.

Nutrition:

Calories: 313 Fat: 7g Protein: 21g Carbs: 21g

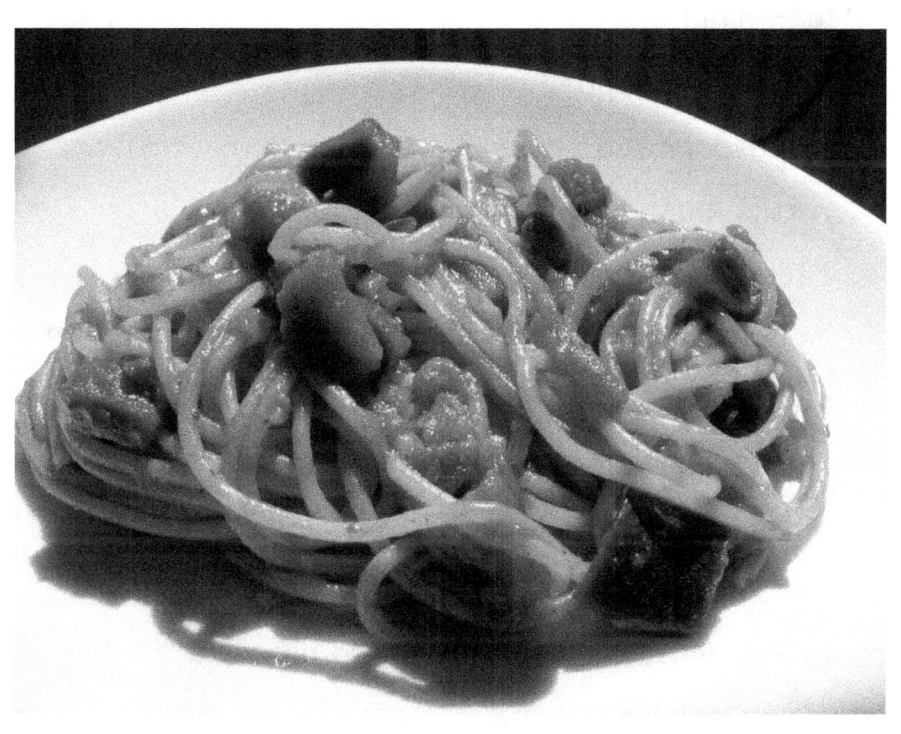

20 Minutes Vegetarian Pasta

Preparation Time: 5 minutes

Cooking Time: 16 minutes

Servings: 4

Ingredients:

3 shallots, chopped

¼ teaspoon red pepper flakes

¼ cup vegan parmesan cheese

2 tbsp olive oil

2 garlic cloves, minced 8-oz. spinach leaves

8-oz. linguine pasta 1 pinch salt

1 pinch black pepper

Directions:

1. Boil water in a pot and add pasta.

2. Cook for about 6 minutes and drain the pasta in a colander.

3. Put oil in a pan and add the shallots.

4. Cook for about 5 minutes until soft and caramelized, and stir in the spinach, garlic, red pepper flakes, salt, and black pepper.

5. Cook for about 5 minutes and add pasta and 2 spoons of pasta water.

6. Stir in the parmesan cheese and dish out in a bowl to serve.

Nutrition:

Calories: 284 Fat: 18g Protein: 19g Carbs: 15g Fiber: 4g

Creamy Vegan Pumpkin Pasta

Preparation Time: 15 minutes

Cooking Time: 5 minutes

Servings: 6

Ingredients:

1 tablespoon olive oil

1 cup raw cashews, drained and rinsed 12 oz. dried penne pasta

1 cup pumpkin puree, canned

1 cup almond milk,

3 garlic cloves

¼ teaspoon ground nutmeg Fresh parsley, for garnish 1 tablespoon lemon juice

¾ teaspoon salt

1 tablespoon fresh sage, chopped

Directions:

1. Make pasta.

2. Cook as the package directions say and drain the pasta into a colander.

3. Dish out the pasta in a large serving bowl and add a dash of olive oil to prevent sticking.

4. Put the pumpkin, cashews, milk, lemon juice, garlic, salt, and nutmeg into the food processor and blend until smooth.

5. Stir in the sauce and sage over the pasta and toss to coat well.

6. Garnish with fresh parsley and dish out to serve hot.

Nutrition:

Calories: 431 Fat: 21g Protein: 25g Carbs: 15g Fiber: 5g

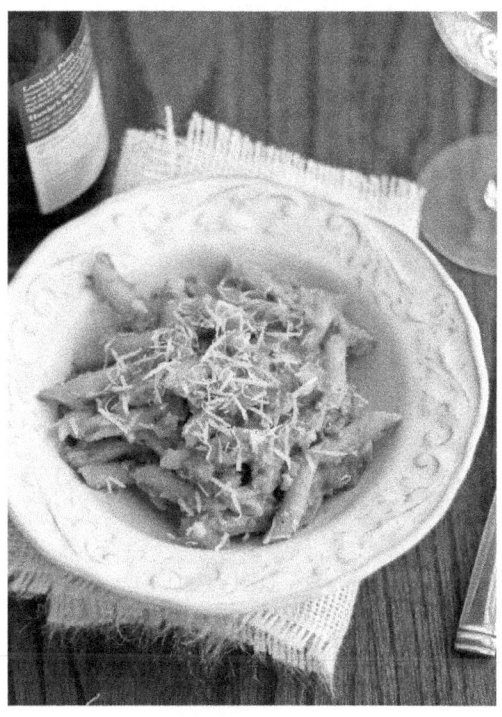

Loaded Creamy Vegan Pesto Pasta

Preparation Time: 15 minutes

Cooking Time: 10 minutes

Servings: 6

Ingredients:

¼ onion, finely chopped 8 romaine lettuce leaves

1 celery stalk, thinly sliced

½ cup blue cheese, crumbled

1 tablespoon olive oil, plus a dash

1 cup almond milk, unflavored and unsweetened

½ cup vegan pesto

1 cup chickpeas, cooked

1 cup fresh arugula, packed 2 tablespoons lemon juice

Salt and black pepper, to taste 6-oz. orecchiette pasta, dried 1 cup full-fat coconut milk

2 tablespoons whole wheat flour 1½ cups cherry tomatoes, halved

½ cup Kalamata olives halved

Red pepper flakes, to taste

Directions:

1. Make pasta.

2. Cook as the package directions say and drain the pasta into a colander.

3. Dish out the pasta in a large serving bowl and add a dash of olive oil to prevent sticking.

4. Put oil in a large pan and whisk in the flour.

5. Cook for about 4 minutes until the mixture begins to smell nutty, and stir in the coconut milk and almond milk.

6. Let the sauce simmer for about 2 minutes and add the chickpeas, olives, and arugula.

7. Stir well and season with lemon juice, red pepper flakes, salt, and black pepper.

8. Dish out into plates and serve hot.

Nutrition:

Calories: 420 Fat: 10g Protein: 31g Carbs: 19g Fiber: 9g

Mediterranean Pizza

Preparation Time: 5 Minutes

Cooking Time: 25 Minutes

Servings: 2

Ingredients:

Cheesy sprinkle (4 Tablespoon.) Classic hummus (.5 c.)

Pizza crusts (Olive oil

Chopped olives (2 Tablespoon.) Halved cherry tomatoes (1 c.)

Sliced red onion Sliced zucchini

Directions:

1. Turn on the oven to 400 degrees. Sprinkle the vegetables on the salt and oil and toss them around.

2. Layout the two crusts on a baking tray and spread half the hummus on each one.

3. Top with the vegetable mixture and some of the cheesy mixture before adding to the oven.

4. After 20 minutes, take these out and then serve.

Nutrition: Calories: 500 Carbs: 58g Fat: 25g Protein: 19g

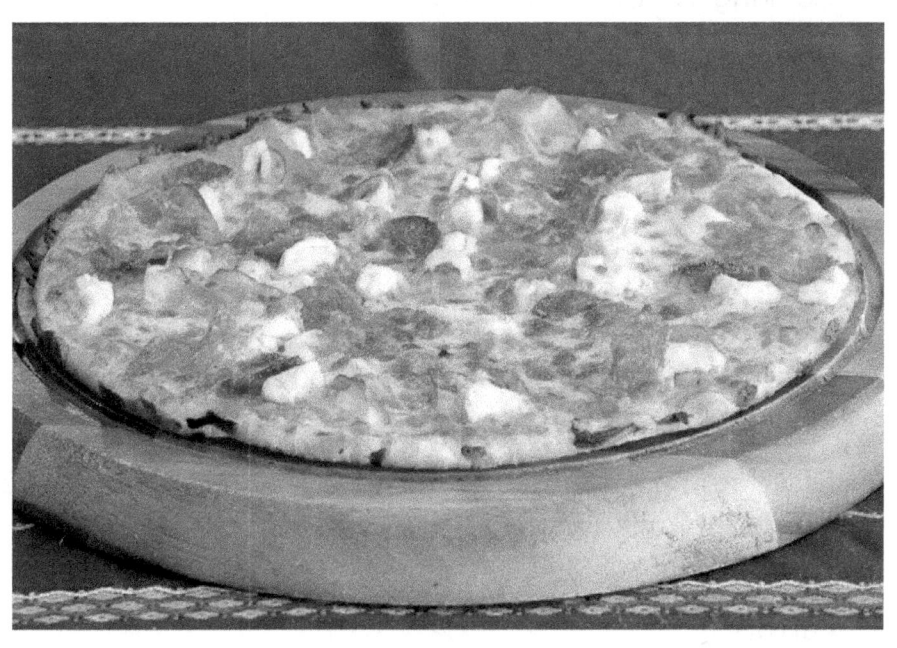

Red Lentil and Chickpea Bowl

Preparation Time: 5 Minutes

Cooking Time: 25 Minutes

Servings: 4

Ingredients:

Salt (1 teaspoon.)

Curry powder (.5 teaspoon.)

Garam masala seasoning (2 teaspoons.) Drained chickpeas (15 oz.)

Diced Roma tomatoes Water (1 c.) Vegetable broth (2 c.) Vegan milk (1 c.)

Dried red lentils (1.5 c.) Diced onion (.5 c.) Chopped carrots (

Directions:

1. To start this recipe, take out a pot and start boiling some water and carrots on the stove. After 5 minutes, you can drain these and set them to one side.

2. As the carrots are boiling, you can heat a bit of oil in a frying pan and cook the onion for a bit. It will take about ten minutes.

3. In a big pan, add in the chickpeas, carrots, milk, water, vegetable broth, lentils, and onion, along with the seasonings and spices.

5. After twenty minutes of cooking, you can take it off the heat before serving and enjoying it.

Nutrition: Calories: 189 Carbs: 22g Fat: 11g Protein: 16g

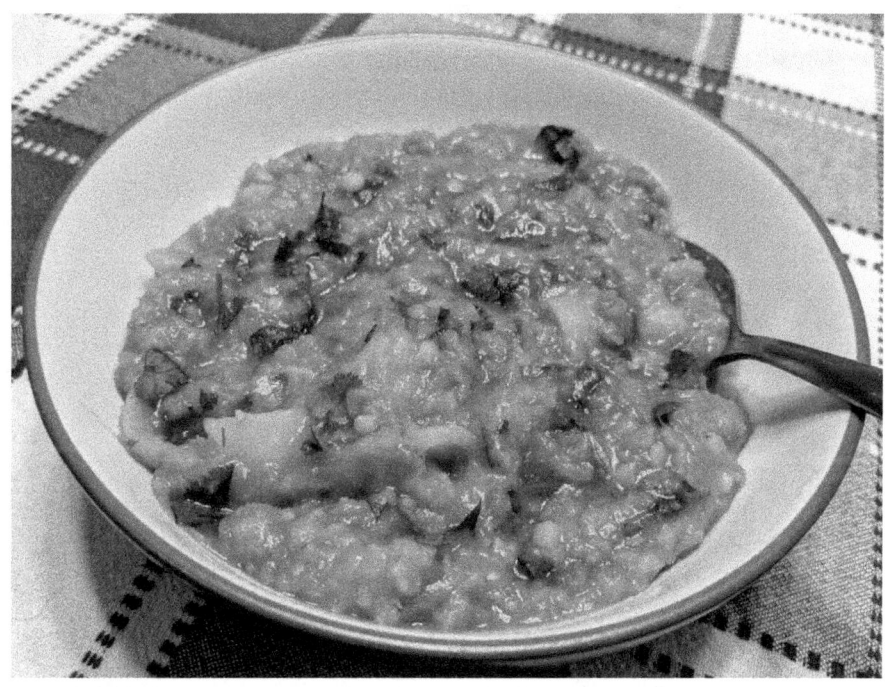

Curry Wraps

Preparation Time: 5 Minutes

Cooking Time: 22 Minutes

Servings: 5

Ingredients:

Chapatis (8)

Sliced garlic cloves Sliced onions

Olive oil (2 Tablespoon.)

Tandoori curry paste (2 Tablespoon.) Cubed tofu (600g)

Mint sauce (3 Tbs.) Yogurt (4 Tablespoon.)

Shredded red cabbage head Quartered lime

Directions:

1.   We can start this out by taking out a bowl and mix the yogurt, cabbage, and mint sauce, then set it to the side.

2.   Toss the tofu and the tandoori paste into a frying pan with some of the oil. Then cook this for a bit on each side to make it all golden brown. Take out of the heat when you are done with this.

3.   Next, we can add the garlic and onions into the same pan and cook

Those for a bit. After ten minutes, add the tofu back in and cook a bit longer.

4. Heat the chapatis using the Directions: on the package and then fill them up with the tandoori tofu and the sauce you made. Serve with the lime quarters.

Nutrition: Calories: 211 Carbs: 22g Fat: 7g Protein: 19g

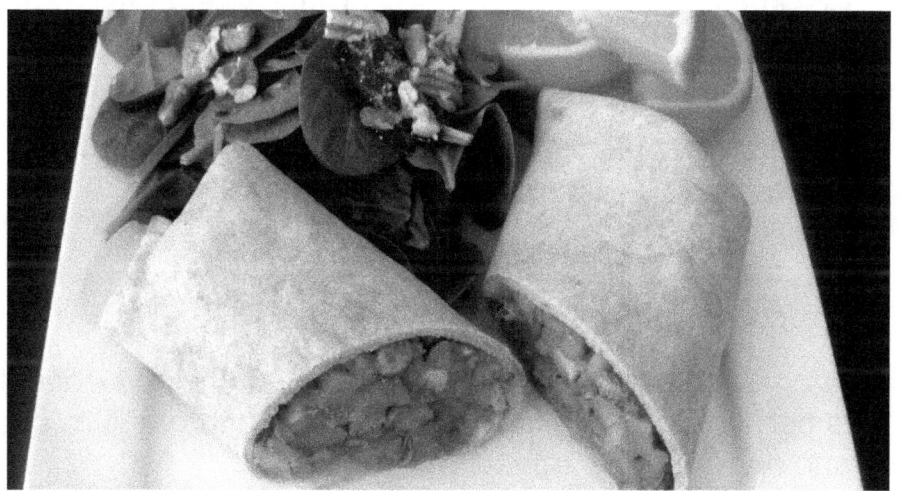

One Pan Spicy Rice

Preparation Time: 5 Minutes

Cooking Time: 25 Minutes

Servings: 5

Ingredients:

Yogurt to serve

Cashew nuts (1 handful) Spinach (2 c.)

Raisins (1 handful)

Chickpeas, rinsed and drained (15 oz.) Vegetable stock (2 c.)

Basmati rice, rinsed (1.5 c.) Curry paste (2 Tablespoons.) Crushed garlic cloves 9 Sunflower oil (1 Tablespoon.)

Directions:

1. Take out a pan and heat some oil inside. When it is hot, you can add in the curry paste and garlic to cook and heat up for a minute.

2. When this is done, add the pepper, salt, chickpeas, raisins, vegetable stock, and rice into the pan and stir it around well.

3. Reduce the heat for a bit and let this cook. After 15 minutes, all of the liquid should be gone, and the

rice should be tender. Add the cashew nuts and the spinach as well.

4.   Serve with some of the natural yogurts and enjoy it.

Nutrition: Calories: 170 Carbs: 16g Fat: 2g Protein: 5g

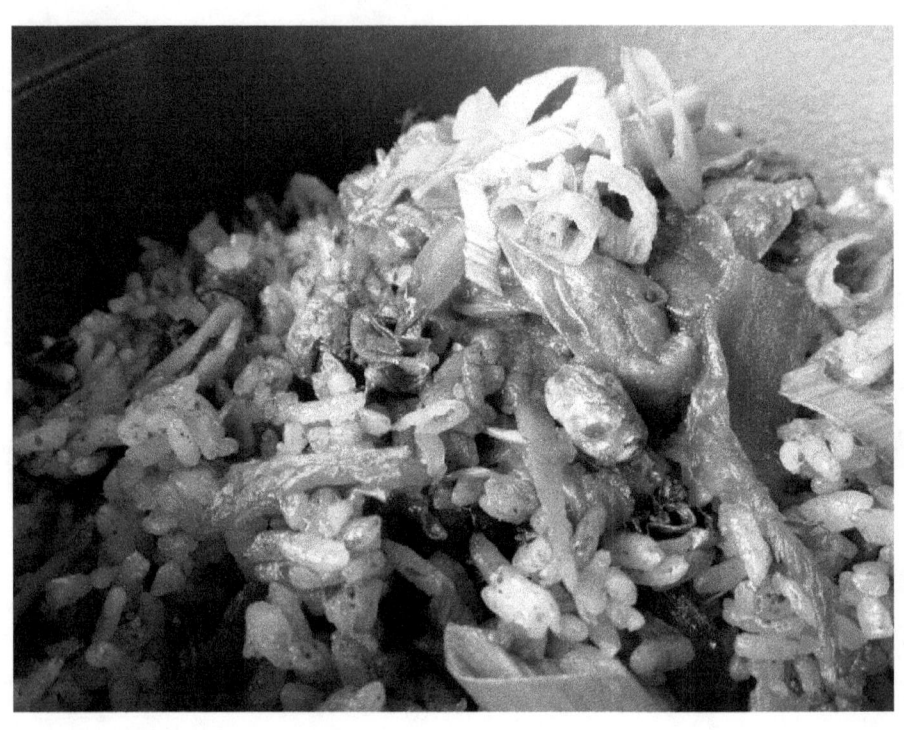

www.ingramcontent.com/pod-product-compliance
Lightning Source LLC
Chambersburg PA
CBHW070722030426
42336CB00013B/1896